ANNIHILATE

ACNE

NOW,

NATURALLY

NICK DELGADO, FACN, ABAAHP, PHD

Annihilate Acne Now, Naturally
By Nick Delgado, ABAAHP, PhD
© 2015 by Nick Delgado

Published by
Health Wellness Studios Inc.
160 Greentree Dr. # 101
Dover, DE 19904

ISBN: 978-0-9962196-0-0

Printed in the United States of America

This book is not intended to provide medical advice or to take the place of medical advice and treatment from your personal physician. Readers are advised to consult their own doctors or other qualified health professionals regarding the treatment of their medical problems. Neither the publisher nor the authors take any responsibility for any possible consequences from any treatment, action or application of medicine, supplement, herb, or preparation to any person reading or following information in this book. If readers are taking prescription medications, again, they should consult with their physicians and not take themselves off medicines to start supplementations or a nutrition program without proper supervision of a physician.

CONTENTS

FOREWORD

By Fran Kerr, author and acne coach
Annihilate Acne Now, Naturally is an important book that needed to be written. From the date of writing this foreword, I have been working in the natural treatment of acne for over eight years. In my opinion, throughout that duration of time, nothing has revolutionized the healing of acne as quickly and as effectively as Dr. Nick Delgado's products.

There was always one piece of the puzzle missing in the "old" way of treating acne naturally and holistically. I personally, along with many men and women I consulted with, were working hard to keep our skin clear. We were striving to be the healthiest people in the world; we were trying our hardest to do everything right, but any minor slip up in our holistic routine would mean yet another acne breakout. What a stressful way to maintain clear skin! It wasn't until the discovery of Estro Block®, and how well it really does *annihilate* acne, that I saw complete and permanent healing in my own skin and in the skin of many others.

And since the creation of Estro Block®, Dr. Nick Delgado has released a range of natural products that make it even easier to completely heal acne.

I am grateful for Dr. Nick Delgado's creativity and dedication to formulating a natural solution for men and women of all ages to get final control of their acne problem. So, read on and be guided into a life *free of acne.*

In the natural treatment of acne it is essential to uncover the root cause of the problem by answering this question: What imbalance in the body is creating acne?

Conventional acne treatments are what I call *bandaid treatments* because they often only fix the problem at the surface level, often leaving the root cause of the acne still present. Either the acne returns once conventional treatment is discontinued (often worse than it originally was), or the imbalance in the body manifests itself by causing other health problems.

So as you can see, the absolute best way to treat acne is with consideration to two very important things:

1. Get to the root cause of the acne and heal it.
2. Work out that cause and prevent it from happening again.

The first is relatively easy to accomplish with the help of Dr. Nick Delgado's products. The second is trickier. I encourage you the reader, having found your way to this book, to delve into the reasons why that imbalance happened in your body in the first place. It could be as simple as going through puberty or coming off the birth control pill for women. But, and this is very important for adult men and women with acne, it could also be caused by chronic stress or emotional issues.

You may not agree with me right now, but having acne-prone skin is a blessing in disguise because it is such a clear indication your body is not in balance. When I get acne, for example, I know that my body is warning me of a problem. It could be as simple as a healing crisis from a detox, or it could be a hormonal imbalance, excess stress in my life, or diet choices I've made that aren't good for my body. We get acne for a reason and there is always a way to heal it.

If there is one message you need to remember from reading this foreword, it is that you will heal your acne, and heal it permanently. You will not have to deal with any level of acne for the rest of your life and *you do not have to take or use chemicals to heal it*! We now have the best natural tools available to us to get to the root cause of your acne and to heal it completely.

Dr. Nick Delgado's Estro Block in combination wiith LivDetox is a highly effective method of getting to the root cause of your acne and healing from it. I personally still use his products to treat my own hormonal imbalances, and recommend his products to my clients daily. I have witnessed so much relief and joy from clients who have finally reached the point of completely clear skin. I am incredibly grateful that Dr. Delgado created these products and made them available to use.

Just remember, healing from acne is often more involved than taking a pill. You will need to accompany your supplementation with diet changes, relaxation techniques, drinking plenty of good quality water every day, regular exercising, and building your sense of self love or releasing stored up emotions.

I wish you all the best on your journey to clear skin.

INTRODUCTION

My Story: Why I wrote Annihilate Acne Now, Naturally

My motivation for me writing this book on supporting healthy skin began at the age of 13 to 15 when my face started to break out. I remember big pimples that I looked at in the mirror with disgust. When I attempted to get rid of them by popping them and picking at them, they would get worse, angry looking, and bloody red. Since young men "don't wear make-up" I felt embarrassed to go to school. I didn't want to look as if I had been in a fight every night.

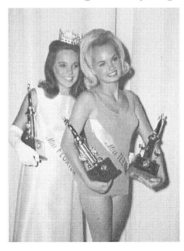

I remember searching for a solution. As Henry Ford says in one of my favorite quotes, "Don't find fault, find solutions." My mother worked days and my father worked nights. My sister Susie and I had the run of the house. I spent a lot of time watching television the year Robert Kennedy and Martin Luther King Jr. were assassinated and the women's liberation movement was building up. As I flipped through a few channels, CBS to NBC to ABC, a live broadcast of shrieking women's liberation protestors attracted my attention. They were protesting the 1969 I Miss America pageant being held. The winner, Judy Ford, Miss Illinois, who won the talent competition performing on a trampoline, said one of her beauty secrets was to rinse her face with purified water every day and night.

When I washed with soap and regular tap water, my face would break out. However, when I tried Miss America's suggestion, rinsing my face with purified bottled water after soaping up, I saw an improvement. The pure clean water helped my face look better.

I also noticed if I went to the beach my skin tanned easily, drying up the oils, and by the next day I had fewer pimples or blackheads. I had no idea at that time why the UV light of the sun dried up sebaceous glands and the purified water reduced the bacteria on my skin and reduced acne. Nor did I realize that my meat- and dairy-based diet would have a profound effect on altering my natural hormones and my skin.

Unfortunately these techniques, using purified water on my face and sun tanning to prevent acne, were not enough. My skin problem continued to haunt me. When I was a freshman in high school, my friend Scott was trying to get into Hollywood and had an extra ticket to see the John Strong show. Audience members were encouraged to ask rehearsed questions of the host.

An agent saw me and invited me to appear on the Dinah Shore Show and Dick Clark's American Bandstand.

I took a few dance lessons and felt energized and confident as I danced in front of the cameras.

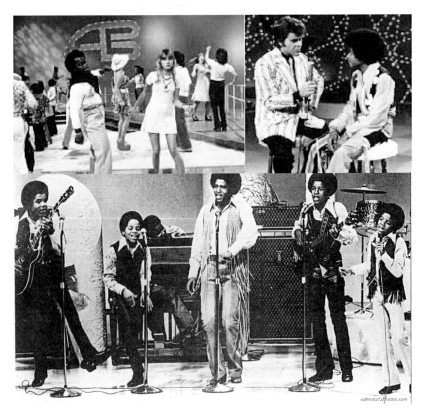

I was on a live set with incredible groups such as The Jackson Five and Steppenwolf.

I was surrounded by the beautiful "Hollywood types" every weekend and the teenage dancers took pride in their youthful healthy look.

We taped several shows on the weekend. We brought several changes of clothes so we looked like we were appearing on different days.

My appearances on American Bandstand were exciting and fun but I felt extremely self-conscious if I had a breakout. One day I looked in the mirror and was so embarrassed that I stopped going to Hollywood auditions and American Bandstand. I normally had an outgoing personality but because of my skin, I was too self-conscious to continue.

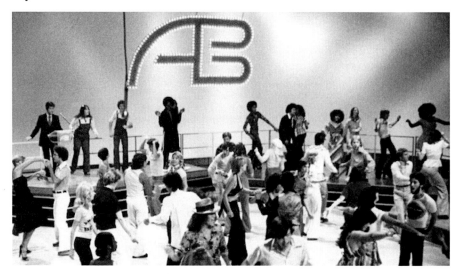

Today I wonder how many young people have had similar experiences that have hindered or prevented them from reaching their goals and dreams in life.

When I was 16 my hormone levels began to change even more. It was football season. After just a few weeks of practicing with the team, I began noticing blackheads and pimples forming where I wore the chin guard of my helmet. To make matters worse, I was expected to gain weight in order to play on the varsity team.

As I lifted weights and ate more protein; meat, cheese omelets, and raw eggs, I did gain weight.

But my skin looked worse.

As my skin went through phases from clear to having breakouts, another more serious health threat developed. My blood pressure shot up so high that the school nurse asked me to come to her office to measure it each month. My doctor told me to reduce stress, relax, and stop eating salt, which I did. I also rarely ate any food with added sugar. My blood pressure didn't change. I was perplexed. Here I was, on the American Diet, the best diet money could buy, high in meat and egg proteins. What I didn't realize was that these foods were high in fat.

At the age of 21 I was put on blood pressure medications. At the age of 22 I suffered my first TIA, (transient ischemic attack) a small stroke, while on hypertensive medications. I was shocked. I now feared for my life. The doctors could not explain why I had such high blood pressure. My first son, Jason, was born and I did not think I would live to see him grow up.

USC, Rancho Los Amigos had accepted me as a graduate student in physical therapy where I worked mostly with stroke victims. It was depressing that after months of rehabilitation these patients often would have another stroke.

After six months I transferred back to the main campus at USC to work toward my newest interest, psychology, to find out what motivates people. I also learned about Nathan Pritikin and the Longevity Center plan to reverse heart disease `and high blood pressure.

When I read Pritikin's book *Live Longer Now,* I finally understood why I had high blood pressure and how my diet was also related to my acne.

By following the Pritikin diet, in only 30 days my blood pressure was reduced to normal and after six months I had lost 50 pounds of excess body fat. I noticed my skin looked better than it ever had. I ate fresh vegetables, fruit, brown rice, beans, and potatoes without butter. I ate no dairy products and no oil. I ate lean meat, chicken, or fish about once a week.

The change in diet was the miracle I had been searching for. This dramatic improvement and my increased energy motivated me to work out with weights, run on the beach and get into super shape. I felt better than I ever had in my entire life.

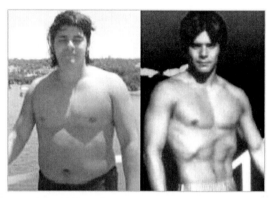

BEFORE   AFTER

I heard that Nathan Pritikin was going to speak in Pasadena California. Nathan had appeared earlier that year on a positive report by 60 minutes and was highly respected by William Castelli, M.D., organizer of the famous Framingham Study. I made sure to go. His lecture set off my fascination with natural healing and optimum performance. Pritikin invited me to work with him in Santa Monica, California at the Longevity Center.

Nathan Pritikin was a scientist, engineer and researcher who had reviewed medical literature. He mentored me on how to present health lectures, treated me like a son and gave me access to all of his abstracts and research.

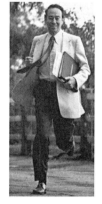

Nathan Pritikin loved to run and I enjoyed running with him. After our workout I would have long discussions with Nathan about research on health longevity. I became director of the Pritikin Better Health Program where I had the privilege of teaching thousands of students at education lectures and workshops.

In 1982 I founded Delgado Medical and began forming programs with doctors to educate the public on good health.

In early 1989 I went to one of the first American Academy of Anti-Aging Medicine conferences held in Las Vegas to learn about balancing hormones. This was the beginning of an incredible opportunity to learn a vast amount of information about how hormones and biochemistry relate to metabolism.

It was at the Las Vegas conferences of 2008 when I was teaching about hormones and metabolism that I met Ray Sahelian, M.D., nutrition expert and author of several books.

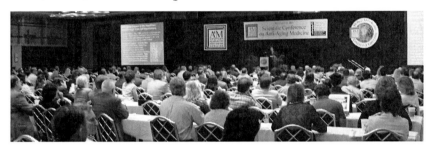

Ray came up to introduce himself and complimented me on my lecture presentation. I will never forget seeing his face

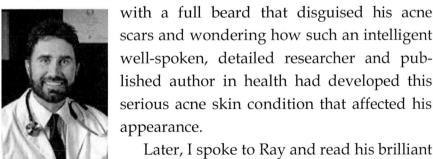

with a full beard that disguised his acne scars and wondering how such an intelligent well-spoken, detailed researcher and published author in health had developed this serious acne skin condition that affected his appearance.

Later, I spoke to Ray and read his brilliant articles regarding acne. He perused integrative natural healing methods combined with his medical training as a result of his severe skin condition. Similarly, this intractable acne and my related health problems were what had led me to search for natural and innovative solutions.

Dr. Ray Sahelian did not find the answers in his medical training.

He, as I, had to go beyond traditional education to make observations to better understand the body's inflammatory response mechanisms. This inflammatory and hormonal disorder called acne can be present in nearly 80% of people exposed to the Western diet and lifestyle. This skin condition, which can first appear during adolescence and worsen during hormonal changes, is influenced by several factors including estrogen and androgen metabolism.

Later, I studied estrogen metabolism and discovered how estrogen dominance could cause drastic changes in androgens in both men and woman. I observed that these hormonal imbalances in estrogen metabolism could cause or worsen acne.

I researched and created natural hormonal modulating products in late 1998 to help restore balance to the body, reduce obesity, and reduce the risk of hormonally related breast cancer in women and prostate cancer in men. At that time I had no idea that supplements combined with lifestyle improvements could also help reduce and annihilate acne naturally.

I wrote several research articles and abstracts for doctors including one called "Estrogen: a Male Toxin?" This was published in the 2003 Anti-Aging Medical News and the Anti-Aging Medical Therapeutics for medical doctors and scientists to understand the complexity of hormones, lifestyle and its relationship to our health.

In 2001, I wrote a book called *Grow Young and Slim* about all of my research and findings regarding hormones, natural diet, exercise, fitness.

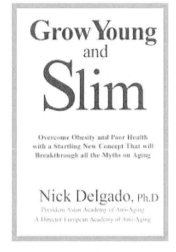

Grow Young
and
Slim

Overcome Obesity and Poor Health with a Startling New Concept That will Breakthrough all the Myths on Aging

Nick Delgado, Ph.D
President Asian Academy of Anti-Aging
A Director European Academy of Anti-Aging

I began hearing from more and more doctors who were using the products I had created with good results, directly related to improvements in hormonal balance. They had observed reductions in body fat and improvements in the skin. I also was surprised to make the clinical observation that young girls and young men, and even women in their early forties had cleared up their skin using our protocols. In some cases their skin had cleared up using products I had created, including specific supplements referred to in the Appendices, without a change in diet or lifestyle. I shared these findings with clients, friends, and relatives, and they too achieved excellent results. It's true that a good word can spread fast, and in this day of the Internet, with bloggers like Fran Kerr of *High on Health*, Tracy Raftl of *The Love Vitamin*, and other forum leaders, people all over the world were hearing about our success helping those with hormonal related skin conditions.

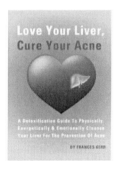

I think what motivated and touched me the most was meeting these individuals and hearing their stories of success. I met many young women and men struggling with a life-long battle with acne. Some of these clients were being exposed to drug therapies with the risk of horrible side effects. Those who tried our natural approach to balance their hormones experienced rapid results. On Facebook, Instagram, or a blog, they would share their heartbreaking stories of embarrassment, attempts to disappear from social life, and then their incredible transformation with before and after pictures and the excitement of solving this seemingly insurmountable personal challenge of their hygiene and its effect on self-esteem. This led me to write this book, *Annihilate Acne Now, Naturally*, as a complete solution.

The Delgado Protocol offers a plan to annihilate acne while assisting you and your family to live a better quality life.

Chapter 1

THE CAUSES OF ACNE

Acne affects over 50 million Americans, with 80% of all people developing acne at some time during their life. Acne treatments cost in excess of $2.2 billion in the United States in 2004.

Why is acne such a large problem in our society? What can people do to get to the cause of the problem without using bandaid treatments such as drugs, antibiotics, and birth control pills? I strongly believe that such treatments are like taking a sledge hammer to swat an ant. They are excessive and can often cause further damage.

In truth, acne is something that should first be addressed with modifications in lifestyle and the proper use of supplements to deal with this global problem.

I will say right in the beginning that there is no one single solution for everyone, and anyone who promises you a quick fix cure to this complex problem is not sharing the full story with you. I will say, however, that a majority of the problems relate directly or indirectly to hormonal imbalances.

Let me first explain my hypothesis and discoveries related to estrogen dominance and its powerful effects on androgens and your skin.

Contrary to common perception, Estrogen is more than just estradiol, estriol, and estrone that most doctors measure in a blood test. There are over 40 different estrogen metabolites! These hormones go through a cascade and change throughout the body, depending on your diet, your exercise, and your emotions. How well do you feel you manage your diet, exercise, and emotions?

Hormonal imbalances are the reason a majority (over 80%) of teenagers age 13 to 19 and young adults age 20 to 25, and an equally shocking high percentage of adults develop acne.

Other contributors to acne and the overall health of your skin include exposure to toxins and how well your liver processes the chemicals. Unfortunately, some people have an amazingly high predisposition to develop acne.

The origin of acne is a complex and often a puzzling issue. Over the past 25 years, I have had to explain the multipart and intertwined hormonal system and its effect on acne to many of my clients. I found that it is best understood by the following story that I will call "The House of Hormones." The characters living in this house include good brothers and sisters, bad brothers and sisters, and a surprising hero.

In this house of hormones, various lifestyles, diets, ands genetic makeups causes many individuals to develop excessive amounts of an androgen called dihydrotestosterone or DHT. DHT acts like the big protective brother. As it builds up in the skin DHT causes an overstimulation of the sebaceous glands (excessive oil secretion onto the surface of the skin,) which can cause acne.

DHT should never be completely to blame nor should it be eliminated because it is necessary. In men, DHT resides in and nourishes the prostate. DHT in women is necessary because it attaches to the hair follicles to provide additional hair growth to protect the pubic area. DHT also improves libido and interest in sex.

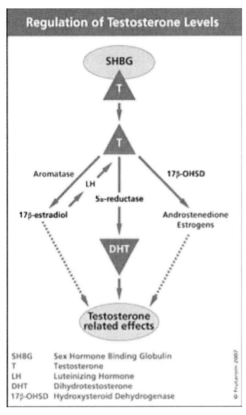

The hormone testosterone and most other androgens will be converted by the enzyme aromatase into estradiol, which eventually turns into either a powerful estrogen called estrone (16aOHE), the "bad sister," or it turns into a "good sister" estrogen called methyoxyestrone (2OHE).

The bad sister can easily overcome or suppress testosterone, "the little brother," yet she can never defeat or overwhelm the "big brother" DHT, because DHT cannot be converted into estradiol.

As the estradiol and estrone increases from external forces such as xenoestrogens, chemicals, estrogen-like hormones, or a fatty diet that further increases the strong "bad sister" estrogens, these sisters gang up on the "little brother" until more of the "big brothers" (DHT) appear to save the day.

In other words, as certain forms of estrogen levels increase in your body, these "bad sisters" exert their harmful effects, causing not only acne but also serious and at times deadly conditions such as breast cancer, fibroids, cysts, ovarian cysts, endometriosis, and obesity.

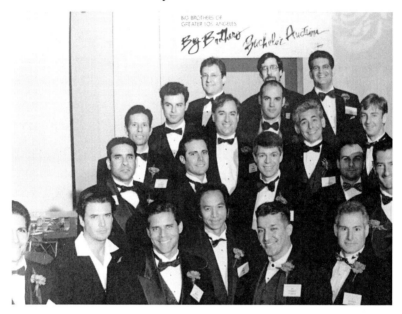

Big Brothers Charity Nick Delgado, PhD, front row, 3rd from left to right & brother, Gilbert Delgado, second row first, behind me

In the winter of 2003 I wrote an in-depth article, "Estrogen, the Male Toxin," published in *Anti-Aging Medical News*. I explained Estrogen dominance in men is caused by the harmful forms of estrogen, the "bad sisters," exerting excessive stimulation of target tissues leading to sexual dysfunction, prostate enlargement, cancer or obesity.

Now the DHT, big brother, arrives because the body, like your house, needs order, so DHT then slows the action of the estrogen. DHT is one of the only androgens potent enough to survive in the presence of concentrated estrogen metabolites. The increased levels of DHT come at price, however, as DHT settles in the skin, causing acne and hair loss in men and women.

Now comes our hero, which we call "DIM" (Di-indolymethane is the phytochemical name) and its related extracts like I3C from cruciferous vegetables. DIM will completely metabolize or push out the "bad sisters" such as 16-Alpha Hydroxyestrone (16aOHE) reducing it to the safe metabolized 2-Hydroyestrone (2OHE). After several weeks the hero DIM does its wonders and the estrogen dominance disappears in the body, restoring order to the house.

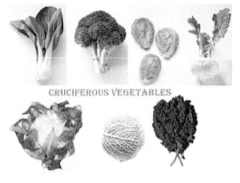

CRUCIFEROUS VEGETABLES

Most doctors up until now have depended on medications to correct this hormone imbalance. Yet we found another method to be equally effective: using natural phytochemicals, herbs, and supplements, and making lifestyle and diet modifications to get rid of the bad sister-estrogens (16aOHE). This allows the "little brother" testosterone to return to a normal level, while the DHT "big brother" can go back to his room and reduce his influence.

There was one more critical step to make the hero effective. We created a very effective way to allow DIM, I3C, and other related phytochemicals to absorb into the tissues where estrogen dominance resides. In this "House of Hormones" I discovered the right combination and assembled it into what I call Estro Block®.

Estro Block® itself comes from natural cruciferous vegetables, like bok choy, broccoli, Brussels sprouts, kohlrabi, cauliflower, savory cabbage, and kale. Concentrates from these food items help to provide natural enzymes. We call them cytochrome enzymes, and these enzymes will help individuals metabolize the bad estrogen forms which have been exerting too much influence on the body, suppressing testosterone, while increasing DHT.

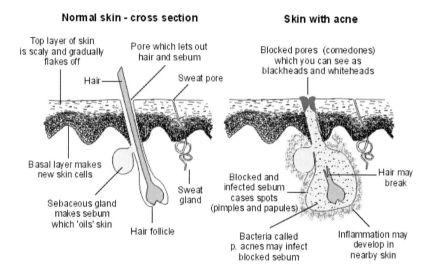

As DHT increases in the skin, this androgen will enhance the growth of bacteria, causing acne, and will overstimulate the sebaceous glands. The solution is not to directly eliminate DHT, but to indirectly gain back control of the estrogen dominance.

Acne may be modified or reduced by focusing on foods that will increase Sex Hormone Binding Globulin (SHBG). These foods include most all vegetables, as well as complex carbohydrates like potatoes and fruit. These foods are naturally low in fat and high fiber. The more raw foods you consume the more you can increase the SHBG.

SHBG will bind to excess androgen (male & female sex hormones that exert androgenic changes). Simultaneously androstenedione will convert into less harmful forms of estrogen called two hydroxyestrone 2OHE. Using supplements rich in cruciferous content will also reduce the levels of androgens.

As the estrogen levels reach their ideal balance with cleansing supplements and a healthier diet, your body supports the proper hormone levels and the acne disappears.

In summary, this illustrates the importance of selecting the right supplements and dosage for your body. Please refer to the Appendix for proper supplements.

These supplements and lifestyle changes provide the liver with the necessary cytochrome enzymes to calm down the "bad sister." When this happens, although this calming effect of your hormones can take a few months, Big Brother (DHT) is no longer needed.

When the "bad sister" estrogen dominance disappears, the "good sisters" can return and play, while the big brother (DHT) returns to his room, because order has been restored; the DHT is reduced to a natural lower level, the good estrogen level is restored, while the testosterone is brought to its normal optimum level as well.

The healthy and proper ratio will be three parts testosterone to one part DHT and less (one tenth) amounts of total estrogens in men.

In women, the ratio will be higher in good estrogen, less total bad estrogen, a big reduction in DHT, and a return to normal levels of testosterone.

Some women should consider estriol cream if tests indicate higher androgen and not enough good estrogen (2OHE), a need for estrogen. Estriol is a safer estrogen, and some doctors feel it provides more benefit with fewer side effects.

Even gentle estriol cream therapy must still be supported with the use of Estro Block® as well as the addition of Adrenal DMG™ with cortisol support to balance potentially higher DHEA levels. The goal here is to prevent too much Estrone

(16aOHE) build up which could be a source indirectly increasing DHT or androstenedione (as explained elsewhere in this book).

We use liver detoxifying supplements (see Appendix) to reduce estradiol--another bad sister that can have too much concentration and exert danger-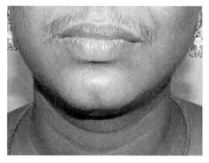ous effects. Excess estradiol can come from the conversion of DHEA, androstenedione, or testosterone. Estriol is the "good sister" along with her good sister 2OHE.

Another cause of acne is polystic ovarian syndrome (PCOS). There appears to be a genetic tendency that increases the hormone testosterone in relationship to other hormones. Some women even develop facial hair.

In this situation, we have worked with doctors who have prescribed bio-identical hormones such as biest cream with Estriol and Estradiol. The added use of supplements such as Estro Block®, combined with a diet rich in fiber, centered around plant based foods, will improve the look of the skin.

Is there a way to take steps to accelerate the healing of your skin? Can you achieve hormonal balance while improving your skin in a series of conscious steps? What if you could learn an effective protocol by reading this book? This book that has taken me 36 years to develop?

Would you?

Chapter 2

THE ESTROGEN CONNECTION

It is increasingly recognized that exposure to environmental, or xenoestrogens, (pronounced zeno-estrogens) is growing. Estrogen-like mimics include pesticides which surround us constantly in the environment. They come from plastic water bottles. They come from certain cosmetics. They even come from some of our fire-retardant bedding. These forms of estrogen absorb into the body and cause chemical havoc.

Next the body tries to excrete these toxic chemicals, which often show up as pimples, and/or acne. That's just one source of additional harmful forms of estrogen in the body.

Another source comes directly from hormones in meat and other foods, although some people believe when you chew up meat and eat it, the digestive juices dissipate the hormones. To an extent, some of these hormones still get through, and we know that people in Argentina and Brazil, where they have a very large cattle industry, eat large amounts of meat that's been fattened up and also injected with hormones.

My visit to Brazil and Argentina in January of 2014 confirmed my suspicion that this culture also tends to have a higher prevalence of acne than non-meat, non-dairy eating groups in Asia or Africa.

It's not just red meat, Dr. Maura McGill and I caution women from consuming chicken (even range feed, hormone free). Dr McGill says estrogen comes from the 3 "P's"-Poultry, Pesticides & plastics. Chicken along with red meat or Fish can cause estrogens to increase. Estrogens' main role is to grow breasts, uterus lining (uterine cyst), and fat cells. Progesterone's role is to be the mother controlling the wild daughter (estrogen). Progesterone and Diindolylmethane DIM (a phyto-chemical) reduces estrogens harmful activities and nurtures healthy activities.

We usually can find the harmful estrogen metabolites in the urine tests. Women can improve their skin by switching from meat, chicken or fish to a plant protein based diet of yams, sweet potatoes, beans, peas, brown rice, vegetables, nuts and seeds (soaked in water to remove the phytate toxins or anti enzyme chemicals), fruits and greens.

A plant based diet is further explained in our book Simply Healthy. Unprocessed, whole foods from plant origins are lower in chemical additives or pesticides than meat, chicken or fish. Because of these massive amounts of hormones and fat in meat, chicken and milk from cows, young girls in these countries now start their menstrual cycles earlier than they ever did in history.

It's frightening, because these hormones cause premature development of breast tissue, ovaries, and an enlarged uterus.

Do you realize at what age a girl would normally begin to menstruate if she were on a healthy whole foods diet? A diet and lifestyle free of added excess fats and oils that overstimulate the hormones, never exposed to these xenoestrogens, and estrogen chemical byproducts? Dr. Hans Diehl, form Loma Linda University researched this question and he states that the average is 16.5 years old!

Confirming this fact are records from Japan in the early 20th century showing young girls did not start their menstrual cycles until about age 16 or 17.

Menstrual periods are now occurring earlier at age 13 in our country and some other countries where meat and dairy products high in fat are the main source of calories.

Periods are further apart, longer, heavier, and more painful when fat intake is high. In addition, menopause (the end of reproductive life) occurs four years earlier (age 46) when on a healthy diet than in those eating a high fat diet.

Worse yet, the rate of acne, heart disease and cancer have increased 10-fold in Japan. Why? The Japanese are exposed to more plastic packaged foods loaded with xeno-estrogens, chemicals, pesticides, and hormones in meat or milk.

In 2006 I traveled to Japan to be a keynote speaker at an Anti-Aging conference. Children in Japan, who eat traditional rice, vegetables, sea vegetables, fruit, and sweet potatoes were slender, fit and a rarely saw a case of acne.

While there, I was amazed and shocked to find KFC and McDonalds restaraunts filled with overweight Japanese teenagers with acne lined up to eat our western fast-food exports. As in the US, many girls now start to menstruate at age 12 to 14.

So, we are comparing the same race (it can't be blamed on genetics) and their menstrual cycle is starting prematurely. It's a worldwide phenomenon now, and here's something that's so often overlooked: The amount of oil or fat in the average person's diet. At the turn of the twentieth century, we know the average person would consume less than 15 to 20 percent of total calories from fat.

They would get fat from whole foods, maybe eating small amounts of nuts, seeds, coconut, avocado, whole mustard seed, and olives. While fruits, vegetables, yams, sweet potatoes, potatoes, legumes, and rice made up most of their diet, which have two to fifteen percent of calories from fat when averaged together.

Now, however, in the Western world we have decided that the principle part of our diet should be high in protein, but what are high protein foods also high in?

Look at meat. Everyone wants marbled, high fat cuts like prime rib, sirloin steak, and the higher the USDA rating of the meat, the higher the fat content. So, when this fat is consumed, whether it comes from unnaturally fattened up beef, or fat from salmon or even chicken, 75% of calories come from fat. When you take the skin off and feel all the grease under the skin in the chicken, you may still have over 40% fat.

We even process foods from Mother Nature. We take fat that comes directly from olives or from coconut, process this food, removing all of the fiber, "cold press it out," and make it into oil. All these oils are so concentrated they are 100% fat. Even extra light virgin olive oil is still 100% fat.

The typical three tablespoons of virgin olive oil mixed into to a salad or cooked as part of stir fry vegetables adds over 42 grams of fat.

Normally the fat is combined with fiber in whole foods such as coconut, avocados, olives or nuts. This fiber slows the absorption and digestion of fat to a rate at which the body can handle it. However, when fats separated from fiber reach the digestive tract, in the gut of the human being, what do you think happens to the fat in its chemical transitions? What hormone growth do you think it stimulates?

Estrogen. In fact, the estrogen levels increase so much that they permeate the entire body. This is one of the major reasons people can develop acne. As people gravitate to a fatty westernized diet, and away from their traditional diet, estrogen levels increase. This also disturbs the androgen balance and the overstimulation of oily skin.

The original Asian food diet was a healthy whole foods diet composed of yams, rice, fruit, and vegetables, with small amounts of fish or meat.

Young people in Asia are now exposed to excess fats and estrogen, which causes estrogen dominance at a very young age. That's why even young boys are developing breasts. Have you ever gone to the beach and seen these young boys who are overweight and already have breast tissue?

Estrogen dominance is permeating our culture. It's everywhere. That's one of the reasons we have adult acne, because our diet is excessively high in fat, high in processed foods, high in sugar, high in chemicals, high in GMOs. The body needs to excrete these harmful chemicals and excess estrogen levels which coexist with "protective androgens" like DHT in the blood and organs, and leavs via the biggest excretion organ in the whole human body.

The skin is the excretion organ at the end point. After the liver tries to detoxify, or get rid of these harmful estrogens triggering abnormally high DHT and androstenedione levels, as well as the toxic chemicals and pesticides, they ooze right to the skin, forming pimples, blackheads, and eventually, acne.

Furthermore, this high fat intake causes an overstimulation of two certain forms of estrogen. One is called estradiol, and the other one, which might be even more harmful, is called estrone -16aOHE.

A young female age 15 to age 35 should have more good estrogen, called estriol, than she does estrone or estradiol, but it's completely opposite in women who have taken birth control pills, because that's mostly estrone. The same is true for women who are taking excessive amounts of estradiol in hormone replacement (that can become more estrone) which is called HRT (synthetic), which is not like natural estriol and estradiol produced in the body at the proper ratio of three to one.

Hormone replacement therapy (HRT) uses synthetic hormones extracted from horse urine and chemically altered in the laboratory. As we build up these levels of estradiol and estrone, we suppress the good estriol levels. The body faces a dilemma. What does it do with all these excess estrogens? They go through another bio-chemical reaction that turns them into one of 40 different estrogen metabolites, and guess what?

Your body has a choice to convert estrogens to a good or a bad form. In the presence of cruciferous vegetables, particularly raw cruciferous vegetables, and whole broccoli, and Brussels sprouts, and cabbage, and in the presence of the correct supplements like Estro Block®, your hormonal balance is restored with an improved ratio of more good (2OHE) than bad (16aOHE) estrogen levels. Just two capsules of Estro Block per day offer a concentrate the equivalent of eating two pounds of raw cruciferous vegetables a day! Do you know anyone who eats two pounds of raw cruciferous vegetables a day?

In the past 16 years, along with a growing number of people around the world, I have eaten a significant amount of raw cruciferous vegetables and taken Estro Block®. With these tools it is easier to get the proper amount of these wonderful phytochemicals to detoxify the harmful estrogens because the body has a choice. The estrogen will either turn into unmetabolized estrogen, called 16 alpha-hydroxyestrone, or 4-methoxyestrone, both of which exert even more damaging effects on the body. The body needs good estrogens like 2-hydroxyesterone and estriol. The damaging effects all come from estrogen dominance that lead to terrible conditions.

We develop acne, endometriosis, and certain forms of breast cancer, uterine cancer, ovarian cancer and obesity. We know that most cancers are estrogen dominant. This leads us to believe, and we're concerned now, that even pancreatic cancer, brain cancer, liver cancer, and bone cancer are all worsened by estrogen dominance.

The good news is that your body has a choice when you take the correct supplements like Estro Block® as suggested in the Appendix. They provide enough of these special cytochrome enzymes to help serve as an inhibitor of biological proteins p450 enzymes. P450 is produced principally in your liver. The function of this P450 enzyme is to convert hormones into more harmful estrogens and more androgens. Estro Block® is the most effective way to stop this conversion and restore balance.

Now remember, androgens would include DHT and androstenedione. So, what we're discovering is if we simply give the body what it needs, even if you're eating a fatty diet, and are exposed to xenoestrogens and chemicals, by giving the body more of these phytochemicals – molecules in plant concentrates – to inhibit the p450 cytochrome enzymes, The selection of the right types and concentrations of phytochemicals will turn these estrogens into a good form of metabolized estrogen called 2-hydroxyestrone, and 2-hydroxyestradiol, and 2-methoxyestradiol. These good estrogens are anti-cancer, anti-acne, anti-obesity, and they actually protect the body according to Dr. Jonathan Wright and other respected researchers (see Appendix 2). Isn't that amazing?

If you have acne all over your body, including your back, face, on your checks, shoulders, arms, legs, buttocks, or pretty much anywhere, then your body and hormones may be out of balance. Did you know that the only place on your body safe from acne is the soles of the feet and palms of the hands where there are no sebaceous glands?

Almost everyone who is eating a Western diet with signs of estrogen dominance needs the Delgado Protocol diet in conjunction with supplements such as Estro Block®, or Estro Block Pro®. I often determine who needs which, based on the severity of their symptoms. If someone is more than 20 pounds overweight, or has severe acne, then what I and a growing number of Anti-Aging doctors often advise is that they should take Estro Block Pro®, which is triple strength.

If they're only five to ten pounds above their ideal bodyweight, and their skin looks pretty good and glowing and they're worried about that occasional pimple, then they should take regular Estro Block®. Or if they're past menopause, (age 50-55) and maybe they're having some mild symptoms of estrogen dominance, then I think Estro Block® regular will be enough. If they choose to take Estro Block Pro® triple strength, perhaps because they are menopausal and no longer cycling, one capsule a day may be enough for them.

Women age 50-55, (particularly if they're overweight, which is a common problem for people past the age of 50 because of hormonal imbalances) may choose to use Estro Block® Pro triple strength; however, they may need some protective good estrogen added to their protocol, taking estriol cream, at a very low dose, using it three weeks out of the month. Even when people are using Estro Block® every day, it's best to take one or two days off from the hormonal estrogen creams each week.

If you are slender, petite and/or over the age of 55, no longer cycling yet your skin is still breaking out, then you can use the new DHT Block™.

My challenge to you is to consider that your skin is dependent on a total approach to wellness. I'd hope that you will continue to follow our direction to achieve healthier skin.

In the next section we will review the benefits of proper daylight and eating foods that are compatible with your genetics and immune system. We will also explore how growth hormones and adrenal functions affect the skin.

Chapter 3

THE SUN, BENEFICIAL HORMONES, NUTRIENTS, AND COMPATIBLE FOOD SELECTION

If you want to improve your diet, take a look at our new book, *Simply Healthy*. This cookbook has over 300 incredible recipes that are gluten free, dairy free, soy free, and low fat. These recipes provide essential fats from whole fat foods, (olives, coconut, nuts, and seeds) but no separated oils and fats and no separated sugars.

Look through the recipes in *Simply Healthy*. I think you'll be astonished. We have Asian recipes, Mexican recipes, Italian, Greek -- all the different cuisines are represented -- and we've spent over 23 years gathering them.

I have been on a quest to locate the healthiest and tastiest recipes. My favorite cookbooks include those by John McDougall, M.D., *Eat to Live* by Joel Fuhrman, M.D., *Going Raw* by Judita Wignall, *The Art of Raw Living Food* by Doreen Virtue and Jenny Ross, *Raw Food for Real People* by Rod Rotondi and . Those books by Brenda Davis, RD, and Vesanto Melina, MS,

RD "*Becoming Raw, Becoming Vegan* and suggestions by Michael Greger, M.D., Dean Ornish M.D., Neal Barnard M.D. Be sure you modify the recipes you find to be gluten free, soy free, and free of added processed oils. Get your essential fats from whole foods and become aware of delayed food allergies and any incompatibility with foods to create a personalized plan. If you would like help, contact us for coaching and advice.

If you're consuming foods that are incompatible with your body, the white blood cells (WBC) have difficulty digesting them. These WBC's ooze out of the skin. Delayed food tests, such as ALLETESS, ALCAT, or Prime can detect foods, spices, and chemicals that cause inflammation.

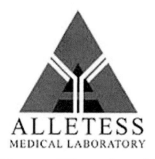

ALLETESS
MEDICAL LABORATORY

The most affordable yet still accurate test is the ALLETESS. This test helps to measure 184 different foods that a person may be sensitive to or incompatible with based on the individual's white blood cell reaction to the foods that they're sensitive to. When the white blood cells break apart, they cause inflammation and/or acne. The skin is a complex excretion organ. Many practitioners believe that blemishes on the skin are toxins being excreted with the immune system going into overdrive, leading to acne. By doing the ALLETESS you will know which foods or spices you are allergic to and you can eliminate just those foods. Wouldn't it be helpful to know which foods and spices are most compatible with you? We can provide you a kit with information on the cost of the test and a requisition to have the blood draw. See Appendix, or go to delgadoprotocol.com

Have you ever noticed that when you go on vacation to a warm, sunny area in the world, your skin seems to improve? Cortisol deficiency can also inflame the skin and sebum glands. Gentle exposure to the sun helps reduce acne because the sun naturally increases healthy adrenal function and cortisol. 500,000 lux of energy comes from the sun, whereas indoor light only allows 50,000 lux of energy.

Although the sun can improve the complexion of your skin, taking Adrenal DMG™ to support healthy adrenal and cortisol levels can further improve complexion. Adrenal DMG™ has glandular extracts for adrenal support. Since glandular extract comes from an animal source, a vegan may choose not to use this product. However, the amount of glandular cortisol is less than five mg per capsule. This small amount will still help support proper glandular function because of the other quality herbs which can also enhance adrenal and immune system function. Adrenal DMG™ also contains important herbs like DMG, which support healthier liver function and healthier more vibrant skin.

Folic acid deficiency can cause acne. To get sufficient amounts of folic acid to help annihilate acne, take the Stay Young™ AM and PM chewable tablets in the morning and capsules in the evening. This product is rich in the most absorbable form of folic acid, 5-Methyl tetrahydrofolate, B12 Methylcobalamin, and natural plant extracts like red spinach nitric oxide burst. These support the release of a potent antioxidant called nitric oxide. There are also many high quality folic acid products available on the market.

There are several factors contributing to acne that can be solved not only naturally, but effectively. It just depends on how motivated a person is to get to the cause of that problem.

Chapter 4

ACNE IS AFFECTED MOST BY WHICH HORMONES?

As you will recall, **I believe testosterone is not the only cause of acne.** Another cause is the imbalance of several hormones, particularly harmful estrogens that cause an increase in androstenedione, which converts into estrone. This combination of androstenedione and estrone influences the stronger androgens such as DHT and free testosterone in the skin, which may affect your skin by making it excessively oily and prone to bacteria proliferation in the presence of excess androgens. The lack of sufficient Sex Hormone Binding Globulin SHBG also plays a role.

Women need testosterone and natural progesterone balanced with good forms of estrogen to reduce fat gain and enjoy a lean, firm body. Women need about one tenth of the testosterone that men need to keep energetic, feel sexy, enhance libido, and prevent mood swings or depression.

The estriol levels in healthy young and older females are typically three times higher than estradiol or estrone, according to Jonathan Wright, MD. This ratio can improve with estriol cream, iodine (15 mg to 30 mg) daily, a whole foods diet and herbs found in Estro Block® & Liv DTox™.

According to our findings and the findings of doctors working with us, this balance can help many of those afflicted with acne to "get to the cause of the problem."

In the early days acne was not known to be connected to abnormally high estrogen levels. The only known connection was that as sex hormone binding globulin (SHBG) increased, the rate of acne decreased. SHBG is a carry protein that transports estrogen and testosterone. Because SHBG binds more tightly to testosterone, a quick, short-term solution was to give women more estrogen from birth control pills to increase the SHBG and suppress acne. Although this solution works, a far more elegant way to solve this complex problem is possible.

Now let's go back to our initial problem of the battle between androgens and harmful forms of estrogen. Another androgen is strong enough to exist in the presence of these powerful estrogens. That androgen is androstenedione. However, as androstenedione has almost estrogen-like activity, it exerts weak androgen activity. Even worse, it will eventually convert into estrone.

This vicious cycle becomes worse if there aren't enough intracellular cytochrome enzymes. Fortunately, **Estro Block®** or **Estro Block Pro®** with **Liver DTox™** delivers the one-two punch to prevent the increase of either "16aOHE estrone" or "4-OH estrone". It is firmly believed by researchers that these chemicals created in the body are highly carcinogenic and may stimulate acne formation, obesity and other severe health conditions.

What if I were to tell you that estrogen molecules exert far more effect on our tissues than does testosterone? Estrogens such as estradiol and 16aOHE estrone have been found to be over **100 times** more potent at the tissue receptor sites than testosterone. Eugene Shippen described this challenge in his book, *Testosterone Syndrome*. These unmetabolized estrogens dominate the weaker testosterone and worsen the skin condition.

These estrogens increase further in women who are overweight, exposed to xenoestrogens from plastics, pesticides and chemicals, or eat a fatty diet.

Female hormone balances can also improve with the addition of progesterone. How is low progesterone related to higher androgens and acne? Progesterone inhibits 5-alpha-reductase, which converts testosterone to DHT. By inhibiting DHT in the skin, you produce less sebum and less chance of acne. Lab tests rarely show elevated levels of DHT or testosterone because the DHT and Free Testosterone concentrate in the skin, not in the blood.

Progesterone in the form of a cream is bio-identical and not synthetic like progestin pills or some birth control pills. Also, some of the progesterone or DHEA may convert into additional estrone, another reason why one should still use supplements such as Estroblock and those listed in the Appendix to clear out any added harmful types of estrogens.

Be sure as a woman, if you are using progesterone (micronized into smaller particles) to use small amounts and take one day off a week and one week off a month. Progesterone in excess can convert to more androstenedione, estrone and 16aOHE estrogen, causing acne and oily skin. So please be careful in monitoring your dosage.

Progesterone in some cases can be used to block the conversion of hormones to DHT, which would reduce acne at very low amounts. Like other natural hormones, progesterone must be used sparingly and in carefully regulated amounts, (during specific times of the female reproductive cycle) based on follow-up blood, urine, and saliva tests.

Doctors who work with us to help our clients are highly trained in anti-aging, employ the use of bio-identical hormones, and use a combination of hormone tests. Urine best measures the various types of estrogens and androgens. Saliva is the easiest and most affordable for a screening and is fine for measuring cortisol. Sex hormone binding proteins are detected only through blood tests. Each has its advantages.

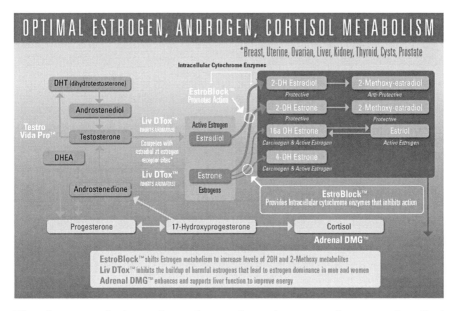

The above graph shows the pathways for estrogen, androgen and cortisol metabolism or breakdown and synthesis of hormones. We have included how Estro Block® (Pro), Liv DTox™, Adrenal DMG™, and Testro Vida Pro™ play a role in balancing hormones to youthful ideal levels.

The most important indicator is the response to interventional endocrinology and supplement therapy. One can use the recommended supplements in the graph above as an additional protective method to minimize the side effects of any hormonal therapy. Hormonal therapy of any kind if not monitored properly, whether it be "natural-Bio Identical", synthetic, used as a cream, pellet or taken orally, can have consequences if not modified by the right combinations of herbal and lifestyle intervention.

Natural hormones for youthful healthy skin

It's inevitable. As we age our skin becomes loose and sags. A gentle rejuvenation approach includes specific amino acids and growth factors, specifically growth hormone. Many of our clients want to know how to maintain youthful skin.

Certain celebrities and athletes have also advocated the use of Growth Hormone (GH), realizing that a majority of this hormone's benefits are rejuvenation and a small aspect is growth. Those taking injectable **Growth Hormone (GH)**, may need to reduce the amount or switch methods to enhance growth factors without over stimulation. Excessive production of sebum (oil) by the skin can be caused during GH treatment. GH improves the uptake of androgens by sebum cells, which produce the skin's oily layer by lowering blood levels of SHBG, thus freeing up androgens that rapidly enter the target cells. The high androgen levels in the sebum cells overstimulate sebum production, which can worsen acne.

History of using natural hormones

There is a long history of using natural hormones to improve the quality of life in humans. In fact, anti-aging medicine was practiced nearly 3,000 years ago by Chinese doctors, who were wise enough to use the urine of young female humans to administer the dried hormones to aging females in their culture. The men were giving the dried hormones from young men's urine with astonishing effectiveness to slow the aging process.

The safety of using these natural hormones was, I believe, also improved by the ancient Asian diet which included more plant-based foods containing nearly 300,000 phytochemicals that provide additional protection and improve the metabolism of hormones in the body, as explained in Chapter 2.

The success of using natural bio-identical hormones in ancient China may have happened because the urine of healthy 15- to 22-year-old young adults contains well over 100 different important hormones that are known to slow the aging process. These hormones from other humans are recognized by the body as bio-identical to achieve safe and effective results.

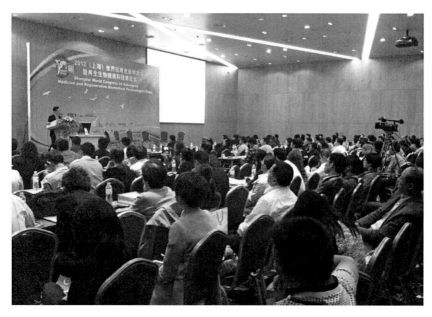

At Delgado Protocol we have chosen to work with the best physicians and health educators trained by the American Academy of Anti-Aging Medicine who utilize more comprehensive approaches to treating acne for each individual.

Doctors working with the Delgado Protocol only use hormones that are bio-identical. Safe, natural sources of hormones from plants like Mexican yams. These plant hormones are then adjusted to be identical to the same hormones your body already produces naturally.

There is a wonderful way in which the body can utilize herbs to support in the production of hormones of youth.

A thorough evaluation by a physician specializing in endocrine balance can help determine which treatment plan is best.

Chapter 5

RESULTS OF IMPROVED DIET & SUPPLEMENT USE

A male client came to see me for a private consult about the acne he was experiencing all over his body. He had the condition for nearly two years before he asked for my help. A dermatologist and several other doctors prescribed medications, antibiotics, and DHT blockers for his acne, all without any improvement.

I gave him some tasty, great recipes and suggested ways to alter his food choices when eating out. For example, instead of always having meat or fish added to his soup, I suggested he replace them with bok choy, broccoli, or yams. I shared my *Simply Healthy Cookbook* approach to eating whole, unprocessed superfoods that are oil-free, dairy-free and fish or meat-free.

I believe the current Okinawan diet is the best as Okinawans are the longest-lived people in the world, have the lowest rates of cancer, have almost no cardiovascular disease, rarely suffer from dementia, and enjoy acne free skin. Okinawans primarily eat yams, vegetables, and fruit, while consuming fish less than twice a month.

I explained to my client that his skin was not only a reflection of the foods he was eating but also the synthetic injections of testosterone he was taking. I felt he could do better using bio-identical pellet testosterone therapy, yet this change alone would not clear his skin of acne. I said to be completely successful, he should try the Delgado Protocol plan for health. If it worked, he would know how to control his acne problem.

My client converted to all natural bio-identical hormones and started using Estro Block®. He took as many as four Estro Block®, one in the morning, one at noon, one in the afternoon, and one at night. His skin condition started to improve. However, because his case was so severe and his lab work showed suspicious hormonal levels in his 24-hour urine test, I urged him to try the type of diet followed by Okinawans. He did, and in less than a month the acne started to disappear; after three months it was completely gone.

He was so excited that when we saw one another at a vegan restaurant, he interrupted a meeting and introduced me to his friends as the health expert who helped him clear up his acne, raising his shirt to prove it.

In February 2014, I was presenting a lecture in Los Angeles to a large audience. During my lecture a tall, good looking man in his 30s, named Ryan (formerly a professional baseball player), stood up and proudly pulled up his shirt to show the whole audience how his back and chest were completely clear of acne after only two months of using Estro Block®.

Now let's review a common intervention for achieving better skin. Let me tell you a story about Sally. She is smart. She wanted to get to the cause of her acne and eliminate it completely.

First she cut back on excess fats in her diet. She immediately started eating more whole super foods. She eliminated processed foods, ate foods with little or no added sugars and fats, and reduced or avoided most meat and dairy products. She exercised daily because that increases SHBG, a binding protein the attaches to excess testosterone or estrogen. She started taking Estro Block®, and using Liv Dtox to accelerate the removal of these harmful estrogens and toxins from her body.

Sally was intent on clearing her skin of acne so she began taking one Liv DTox in the morning and one at night. Some clients have an additional flare up when they are experimenting with what dosage and lifestyle changes will work best for them. For example, a few of Sally's friends had severe cases of acne, so they took three per day, one in the morning, one in the afternoon, and one in the evening. This worked even better for them.

Sally's mom had a challenge with cancer as well as a liver detoxification issue that extended way beyond the acne problem. She started taking four a day, each capsule three hours apart.

Now that Sally, her friends, and her mom are using this combination, enhancing liver function, they're converting bad estrogens into good. The DHT is no longer elevated, decreasing testosterone levels. This is all good, yet a person may have limited liver function to clear all these additional estrogen metabolites trying to leave the body. This is where added B vitamins and improved diet and exercise will improve each person's success.

We measured her lab levels. The DHT reached a balance of one to three ratio to testosterone, while the estrogen reduced to its natural level as compared to DHT. As the estrogen dominance disappeared in Sally, her mom, and Sally's friends, they all noticed a reduction in excess body fat; improved body tone and their acne reduced or disappeared.

These individuals have just enough testosterone for libido and the elimination of cellulite. Testosterone also improves your mood, your ability to think and process in a focused manner, and helps build bone density. Look at the women in our countries who have very poor bone density. They don't have enough testosterone; they have too much bad estrogen. Some doctors give estrogen to build up bone density, not realizing that estrogen builds up soft bone, not the good strong bone the body needs. In some of these cases a women may need to add a small amount of testosterone to build up the bone density while controlling for any additional estrogen conversion by using Estro Block.

A day doesn't go by now without someone, usually a young woman or man in my office, asking me, "How can we spread the word about the Delgado Protocol and the use of your products to help annihilate acne?" This book is the first step in teaching everyone about this comprehensive natural approach.

It takes only a little discipline, because once you break your old habits, you'll never go back. There will be multiple rewards as your start experiencing small success.

If you look at a person who has followed our approach to achieve nice skin and you like what you see, then my protocol is all you may need to achieve good-looking skin. The next section of this book is the most exciting. You will see and read about actual transformations from acne ridden to normal skin.

Appendix 1

REVIEWS ABOUT ESTRO BLOCK® FROM BETWEENTHEKIDS.COM AND PURELYTWINS.COM

Here are examples of how well Estro Block® and lifestyle changes work to clear up acne. These actual cases are for education and cannot be used in place of future clinical research studies. Please, if you are taking any or synthetic hormone therapy for the treatment of acne, have your doctor read the scientific explanation of how to properly guide you in choosing the best natural therapies that are right for you.

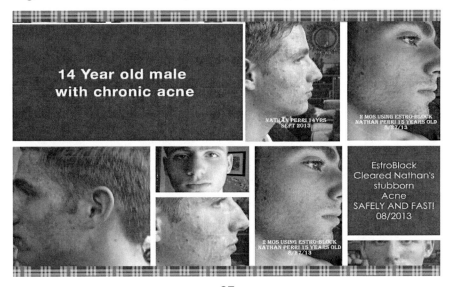

Here is Nathan Perri, who, like other members of his family, was plagued with acne. He shared these untouched photos with us before and after using Estro Block®. As you can see, the results after only two months of using Estro Block® are amazing!

Reviews from blog www.betweenthekids.com

"We recently had the opportunity to review a pretty awesome product, called Estro Block®, that not only helps control acne, but hones in on the cause and promotes overall health and wellness, too. Not only has Kylie noticed healthier skin, but she also says that she noticed that she doesn't have such a big appetite, that her hair has grown faster and she feels great.

"OK so we're talking about estrogen, so this product must be for females only, right? NO. Further from wrong – and I know that for a fact,, because our teenage neighbor was also given a 30-day supply to help improve his skin, and he told me that he has definitely noticed a big difference while taking Estro Block®. Take a look for yourself!"

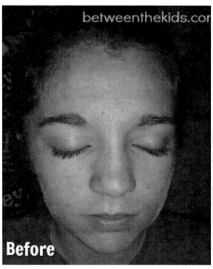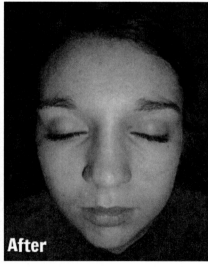

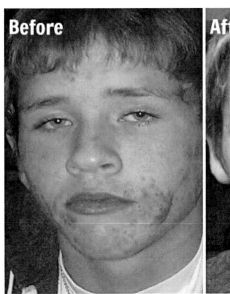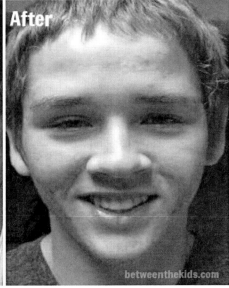

Review from www.purelytwins.com

"A few weeks ago. This was my face before I started taking Estro Block®. As you can see I used to have a lot of hormonal acne on both sides of my face (cheeks, jaw line area)"

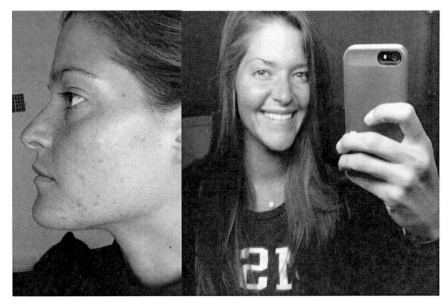

Appendix 2

REVIEWS/TESTIMONIALS

Personal Testimonials

"I appreciate you using my review as Estro Block® has changed my life for the better. Three months prior to this my menstrual cycle was a mess. I would have 10-day periods extremely painful, I'd have to skip work and be miserable. About seven days before I would menstruate I would have horrendous mood swings, crying, depressed, out of control anger. It was a mess. Not only that I had horrible skin to go along with it. I had tried EVERYTHING.

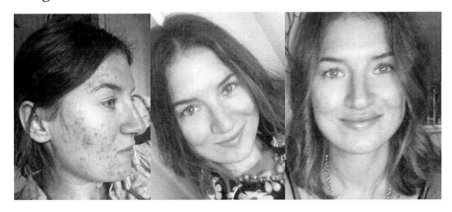

"I tried Cleanses, caveman regimen, Proactiv, tea tree oil, manuka honey, vegan, vegetarian, paleo, meditation, yoga absolutely anything possible. I am in my early twenties and have no idea where this all started. My acne lasted for about seven months and would get more and more severe every day. I would be waking up with 9-12 new pimples a day. I formed very hard cystic ones that would take a week, to two weeks to even subside. I was in pain but mostly absolutely miserable. "I didn't want to be seen in public and I removed all the mirrors in my place because I didn't want to see myself. I found Estro Block® through the love vitamin blog. I immediately purchased a bottle. It made my skin purge drastically. For the first month it made my skin worse than it had ever been. I reached out to Nick Delgado. His helpful team assisted me with dosage and adrenal and cell stabilizer supplements. I started a regimen of taking two pro strength Estro Block®, six adrenal DMG, two cell stabilizers a day. Split up, once in the morning and once in the evening. Then my skin started improving. Day by day I noticed more and more improvement. My skin started lightening up, no more hard lumps around my jaw and chin. My forehead acne completely shut down. My cheeks soreness and bumps subsided. Three months later and my skin looks SO MUCH BETTER! I get maybe one tiny pimple before my period and that's it. Not to mention my menstrual cycle is pristine! It lasts about 5-6 days if that, no cramps, no mood swings, no more hair loss, no more fatigue. I am so thankful as I thought I was doomed forever. I was in such a bad place and scared I had to stay that way forever. Estro Block® has helped me not only on the exterior but interior as well and I couldn't be more thankful!!! I am now taking two pro strength Estro Block®s a day along with six adrenals and two cell stabilizers. I found your account by searching for it. I wanted to see other people's experiences because at one point I wanted to give up on Estro Block® because it was making my skin purge so badly so I wanted to see if others were going through the same thing. I've only been following for almost two months. I find it helpful not only for the testimonies but because it is so positive and there are so many health tips. I also find that I find new friends to follow through the account that are on the same journey as me! Thank you so very much!"

--Marnie Perri

"So good news, I have clear skin for the first time in 13 years. Did I mention I'm on my period right now and this past week it has just been getting progressively better and glowier? I even went off my paleo diet for a few days because I was working long hours on a film set and had to eat the food they offered: donuts and pizza. I thought for sure I would break out but I just came home to healthy, glowy skin, lol. I am kind of in shock. After 13 years of suffering from acne (Age 12-25) I just want to say "That's it? It's over?? Is this a trick??" I still don't believe it. My period is also less painful, less heavy.

"I have been using Estro Block Pro® for about four weeks. I take four pills per day, rather than the two written on the label because I've noticed that it works better for me and the staff said it's safe to take. The first two weeks my skin got worse than it had been for a long time. I had breakouts on my chin, cheeks, and temples. I was moody and my pee was brown every morning. I found it hard to push through because I didn't really know if it was working and the acne was really hard to bear. The third week the breakouts started slowing down, my pee went from dark brown to orange, and the fourth week my skin was clear and my pee was yellow. I honestly didn't expect this to work because after trying so many things, I was used to being disappointed.

"Not sure if everyone goes through this, but I feel kind of ripped off that I suffered deeply with cystic acne for so many years, when there was just a vegetable pill available to fix it. I guess it is a mixture of ecstatic relief and bitterness because I really don't understand why this cystic acne happened to me, it felt like just meaningless suffering that put me over the edge so many times. I can't express the feeling of rubbing my hands over my face and feeling real human skin, without pain, infection and scabbing. I even called my mom and said, 'Wow, my skin color is white, not red.'

"I want to help people find this product, because there are so many men and women whose lives it would change. I am in shock that this exists. I went to my doctor when I started Estro Block® because I had a very rough first two weeks on it. He told me that it was just the way my skin was and that I should give up with the natural remedies and that if it bothered me so much that Accutane was an option. I do believe he was trying to help me, but I find it so frustrating that DIM clearly helps so many people and so few acne sufferers know about it.

"Even worse, I can't believe that I had deep facial infections for half my life due to estrogens caused by pollution and bad nutrition. I had by far the worst acne when at age 14. I decided to become a vegetarian and live on soy meat replacements that are so high in estrogens. My acne went from normal breakouts, to cysts covering my whole face. Soy should be treated as a medicine not a food! It wasn't until I was 19 and quit that ridiculous diet that my acne backed off a bit.

"I've read some reviews where it didn't work for some people. Maybe it doesn't work for everyone, but I also think that some people need to take stronger dosages than what the label says. I've done some Internet research and apparently DIM has been studied a lot and is considered safe in much higher dosages than what the pills include. I have to take four per day which has cleared my skin, and I am considering taking six to see if it will help my anxiety stabilize as I think it is due to hormones. Yeah, it costs more to up your dosage, but I know anyone who has suffered from deforming cysts is willing to pay it. The company is also great as they are there to help you through it and answer all your questions and address your worries. I emailed Rachel a lot (like at least eight emails) and she was able to give me info about other people's experiences and assure me that everything would be okay. I also find their Instagram helpful as it shows before and after images that can help you stay calm if you are going through a bad detox."

-Anna Frank

"I just wanted to write to you guys. I love your products. Especially Estro Block®. I'll take you through my background. I am an Indian and since my teens I had bad acne issues. Always suffered bad cystic acnes throughout and you very well know how frustrating it is to go through that. I never knew that bad eating habits, fat, sugar, toxins, and the environment does play a very important role in making my skin and emotional health worse. My hormones went crazy and I was diagnosed with polycystic ovary syndrome (PCOS). All the doctors had only antibiotics and contraceptives to prescribe. I decided to go holistic by following many blogs and changed my lifestyle. I felt good and reduced weight, but as soon as I ate any sugary food I had big acne on my face. I was always in the fear that I can never eat something I want to once in a blue moon. Somebody recommended Estro Block®. I guess that was Fran Kerr on her blog and as I was taking all the supplements that never helped me I went ahead and ordered that too just a month before my wedding. I started taking six capsules and could see the difference in six days. Now post one year of my marriage I am still having Estro Block® and loved the product and so does my husband who was getting bald at a very early age and also had acne issues can see a big difference. Everyone in my family loves your products. I wish I lived in the US and could work with you so that I can help others too. Whenever you want to open or expand your work do let me know. I would love to help you and work for you. Hope to meet you when I next come to the US. I Love you Nick."

-Lots of love, Sachi

Amazon.com reviews

"I used Estro Block® for my hormonal acne after coming off birth control a few years ago. I had some bad breakouts, especially on my cheeks, jaw line, and chin, and I'd tried everything, you name it - Proactiv, medicated level Sacylic acid, antibiotics, candida cleanses and cutting coffee, sugar, gluten and common allergens, heavy probiotics, anti-fungal, the oil cleansing method...the list goes on. I used Estro Block® with great success for two months and then switched to Source Naturals DIM because it was cheaper and easier to ship where I am currently living - BIGGEST MISTAKE! It actually made my acne so much worse and gave me huge cystic acne in places and sizes like I've never had before. After using it for two weeks I switched back to Estro Block®. I've only been on it one month now but already I have hardly any active acne. I don't believe in miracle products, especially for acne, but if there ever was one THIS IS IT. No side effects at all, in fact my PMS has decreased and I feel more emotionally stable. Highly recommend!!!"

-- Kasandra Bracken, May 28, 2013

"I am ordering my third bottle as I type this because I love it so much. I've been on birth control for the past couple years but was still getting TONS of cystic breakouts, from my nose down. I also decided since that birth control wasn't doing a thing for my acne, I would get off of it after reading 1,000 horror stories about breakouts even worse after getting off. Well, the combination of taking this once in the morning and once at night...sometimes twice in the morning twice at night...eradicated any cystic acne. I am the only person I know who had an easy time getting off of birth control in terms of acne."

-- A. Gordon

"I've had problems with acne since I was a teenager, but when I got into my late 20s the acne intensified into huge, painful sacs all over my face. I did allergy testing, cleaned-up my diet, and had a product routine that I felt worked well, and even though all of these things helped, I was still getting the painful welts on my chin, jawline and cheekbone. I started taking Estro Block® and noticed an improvement within the first week. I've now been taking it for about one and half months and the change is drastic - the acne on my chin, jawline and cheekbone has all but gone away. I'm still getting the occasional pimple here and there, but it's such a dramatic improvement from before that I can't help but be thrilled. As an extra bonus, I've noticed that it's been easier to maintain my weight, and I even have less fat on my legs and butt (i.e., cellulite)! This last part was not something I expected or was looking for, so when I noticed my rear-end looking better I thought I was just seeing things. But lo and behold, my backside is looking better...and this is without changing any other part of my diet or exercise."

-- Julie, February 18, 2014

"I have been 110% pleased and satisfied with both this product and the customer service provided by the staff at Delgado Protocol. I read the reviews here on Amazon and was impressed with other people's results. My results have been awesome. My skin is more beautiful than it has been in months and I've also reduced my weight by 22 lbs. I was so happy with Estro Block Pro Triple Strength® that I also tried and love other products too- Estro Block Cell Stabilizer™, Adrenal DMG™, Lean-n-Fit™, RAD Iodine™. These products all contributed to my improved health, energy, and weight loss. I've had my doctor measure my hormones as was recommended and during the three-month period my levels have improved to youthful levels. I'm 45 years old and have four children ages 11-19. I'm a busy full-time real estate investor who flips houses in Southern California. I'm in the public eye to speak as well as attract investors into my business so my increased energy and more attractive appearance has been hugely beneficial to my career and family. I first saw Dr. Delgado speak at a seminar in San Diego in July 2013, and have since attended many of his classes, events, and symposiums. Both Nick Delgado and his staff have provided powerful, practical, and easy to follow advice to assist me in my health goals. Another aspect of the Delgado Protocol is that he encourages whole foods plant-based diet, rapid fitness, and training the mind to focus on your goals."

-- Health Nut (CA), December 8, 2013

"I can't praise this product enough. Since I wanted to get off of harmful and toxic medications/antibiotics, I tried many other methods in hopes of clearing up some serious (think large and painful) acne. This has been a long and expensive road to recovery… Although I do enjoy keeping a mostly Paleo lifestyle, Estro Block® Triple Strength has been the miracle worker I needed. I've read some reviewers say they noticed a change after three months, but I saw a dramatic difference after only three weeks! I'm on bottle #2 now and every day I am thankful for the changes it has made. After trying other expensive methods with no success, I'll gladly spend $40 a month on a product that truly works."

-- Tara (Greenville, SC), December 11, 2013

"I am a 22-year-old female who has been suffering the past year with adult acne. I went off birth control about eight months ago and ever since then my acne has been worse than ever, especially right around that time of the month. I have seen a dermatologist and even they said my hormones are just through the roof right now. I decided to give these pills a try and it seems to be the magic touch. I was on minocycline for the past two years and that helped a little. Any topical I've

been prescribed just didn't do the trick. I have been on Estro Block® for about two weeks and even my co-workers have noticed a difference in my appearance. My acne is still present, but it's minimum and the bumps are smaller and actually don't hurt anymore. These pills are worth the $30."
— **Mariah (Rochester, MN), November 26, 2013**

"I totally recommend this product! I came across Estro Block® through someone else's testimony on YouTube. I read up on all the information and listened to all the tutorials I could find on Estro Block®. After having no success with allopathic medicine for acne I thought, "I'll have the kids try it." One day after they were taking it, their acne started to calm down and heal, oily skin subsided! I couldn't believe it! My daughter got off spironolactone (suppresses androgen) for the first time in three years! There have been no side effects except one of my boys had a small headache on and off for about a week but nothing since then. I am very excited about the other benefits to Estro Block® as well, but I cannot tell you how much I appreciate Dr. Delgado for formulating the first natural product for the clearing of acne. Hormonal imbalance is one of the number one issues that people are continually seeking answers for. I can't think of one product on the market that is safe and truly effective as Estro Block®."
— **Marnie Perri CPT, NHC, September 26, 2013**

"I have never written a product review before, EVER! I have tried many different products for my acne, which I have had since middle school. I recently stopped my birth control and my acne took on a whole new life of its own. I have been taking Estro Block Pro® for two weeks now. I take one in the morning and one at night. I have noticed my skin clearing up slowly but surely. I am excited to continue to see improvements. I will be posting and updating. No side effects so far. This supplement is worth a try!"

-- **Caitlin Thomas, March 4, 2014**

"Of course when you hear something that sounds too good to be true, it normally is. But this stuff works! I'm 32 and have had cystic acne on my chin for years. I bought this as a last ditch effort to get rid of it. I started taking one pill in the morning and one at night. After a month my acne was much less. Then I decided to take both of them at the same time. That is the miracle trick. No more cystic acne after a week like that. I ran out and didn't order soon enough. Within two days my acne was coming back. So this stuff works for sure. I don't care how much it costs, I feel so much better now!"

-- **Sharon Stump, October 28, 2013**

"I am following up from my previous post because I said I would. I recently posted that I was taking Estro Block® (three pills daily) and it helped but did not cure it. I ran out and decided to try the triple strength and something happened with my package and I didn't receive it until two weeks later. During this time my skin was beginning to break out again. After finally receiving my package I started to take two a day, one in the morning and one and night, let me say this: I have not broken out since then. I think I got one tiny little one that diminished after a day. I have been taking the product for about two weeks and no longer wear foundation to bed because I was embarrassed that my husband would see. I honestly did not think this product would work. It's incredible! I have a clear face which is something I have not been able to say for quite some time. I will post again to keep everyone updated because I am curious how long this will work. Nothing is more embarrassing than hiding your face. Now I don't have to. Please, if the other pills don't work, try triple strength!!"

-- Theresa, March 3, 2014

"The title is not an exaggeration. I have waited months to post this review just to ensure that the results I felt stemmed from this product were applicable. Let's see, I tried this back in early November and it is now February so I think I can post this with some confidence. I have known about Estro Block® and DIM for a long time due to the unseemly amount of research one goes through when trying to divest themselves of acne. I have heard and known about it for years but was 1) wary of it, and 2) didn't not have the money or means to purchase it. So, when I did I first tried just regular old DIM, the Source Naturals brand. It caused me to break out a lot, and I lost a little hope because DIM was a last resort in my long battle to get clear. I gave up on DIM for a few months but then, on reading some more reviews, read that the difference between regular DIM (Source Naturals and others) and Estro Block® is not to be trifled with. I gave Estro Block® a chance. I couldn't be happier. At the time, I had breakouts every day-- anywhere from five to a dozen pimples on my face at a time, often more. Nothing was stopping it. Nothing was helping. When I started Estro Block®, results weren't immediate but it sure as hell was fast in comparison to the years and years of having acne. Within a few weeks my face was clear, and I do mean clear. I did not get another pimple until late December (and I wasn't surprised or upset about it. I was under loads of stress from work and relationships--DIM can't carry the whole load). I have had few pimples in January but I can count them on one hand. I am through-the-roof happy!! Nothing has worked this well! Nothing!"

                                 -- **Tamar Floyd, February 2, 2014**

"The only thing in my 47 years of dealing with hormonal cystic acne that WORKS. If you can think it, I tried it. Then I found this. I won't be without it!!! Give it a month, but you'll see small improvements almost right away."

                                 -- **Laura Howard, March 4, 2014**

"I have been suffering with hormonal acne for over 30 years and have been prescribed all sorts of treatments from the hospital and GP, some worked however they came with unpleasant side effects. Dr. Nick Delgado's team recommended Estro Block Pro® and I haven't looked back! Within a couple of weeks my skin was amazing, people comment how lovely my skin is. Estro Block® is like magic and I'm very happy, confident, and frequently go out with no make-up at all - why cover up beautiful skin! With all the other benefits Estro Block® has to offer - I'm completely converted!"

                                 -- **Mariah Sayer, January 26, 2014**

"After reading lots about Estro Block® and how it can clear up hormonal acne, I decided to order some even though the product is expensive and I had to pay postage and customs charges for the UK. But it was well worth the money. I noticed an instant improvement in my skin (jaw line acne) and I have just completed taking one bottle of pills and my skin is SO much better than it was. The odd stubborn cystic spot is taking a while to disappear, but they are going slowly! All the other spots totally cleared up quite quickly and the red scars are darkening and slowly disappearing. I would definitely recommend Estro Block Pro® to anyone who came off the contraceptive pill (like me), but then their skin just erupted in cystic horrible acne."

-- Chlemsford1 (Essex, UK), December 31, 2013

"So I am 23 years old and my skin is combination but mostly oily. I used to suffer from cystic acne that would swell up half my face if it was in the right spot. I started making jokes that I was in fight club and I couldn't talk about it. I tried to accept it but I was so self-conscious I was about to get off my natural regimen and go to prescriptions. Last year I started to get this weird breakout that could have been hormonal. I was putting lotion and foundation on in layers to cover it up just hoping people wouldn't stand close enough to see it. That was the tip of the iceberg for me because I was constantly looking in the mirror and it was affecting my confidence and comfort, even in my marriage. I started looking into hormonal acne. I found that DIM has helped a lot of people so then I researched that a bit and found Estro Block® from Delgado Protocol. I started taking Triple Strength in September and right away all of the nasty dermatitis-like areas healed. THAT was a relief. I still get sporadic regular pimples that are low grade and quick to heal and I probably get them because I pick at my face. I would recommend this product for anybody who wants to rid themselves of hormonal acne and start clearing their body of toxins. If you're looking for results, this product is WELL worth the price. DP will keep my business."

-- Angela Gowdy (Alaska, US), October 17, 2013

"I been using Estro Block® for three months. This product is awesome. I feel confident taking it because it is safe. It is the only non-chemical product I have found to clear up my skin. I encourage you to educate yourself online and through Dr. Delgado's videos so that you are confident before you take something. I highly recommend this product."

-- **Brandon, September 6, 2013**

"This stuff is amazing! My skin has not been this clear in years. If you have hormonal acne you have to try this stuff. I'm 34, have been struggling with hormonal acne for years, and finally I found a preventative. I am so thankful. I've prayed and prayed to find a solution and my prayers have been answered. I started off with the DIM and the estrogen blocker worked much faster. I am on my second bottle and skin is so much clearer. I'm just waiting for acne marks to disappear. I will continue to use this product so please do not discontinue. I would give it 20 ★★★★★★★★★★★★★★★★★★ ★★★★ if I could. Thank you for changing my life!"

-- **Jennifer, December 7, 2013**

"I came off the birth control pill in May and shortly thereafter I had severe acne. I had very little acne as a teenager. I did have a case of it in my twenties which was treated with Spironolactone prescribed by my dermatologist. I went back to my dermatologist and asked how to clear up my skin and he recommended that I go back on the pill and the Spironolactone. I was cruising the net one day and saw a blog by The Vitamin Lady where she recommends Estro Block® for Adult Hormonal Acne (which is what I'm being told I have). I decided to give the Triple Strength a try. At this point what could I lose? It's been one month and I can tell you my face is 95% cleared up. I have been very happy with the results of the Estro Block®. Also, as a side note, I have gone from a size 9 to a size five in a little over a month's time. I wasn't taking this for weight loss but apparently it has assisted me in this as well. I do eat very healthy but I haven't been a size 5/6 since high school. This is a great product. I will continue to take it."

– **J. Boisjoly (Thomson's Station, TN), December 2, 2013**

"I have had cystic/ hormonal acne for about 10 years. I'm 26 now and I know this product has really worked. I took a little more than the recommended dosage at first just to get a jump start and I could see the light at the end of the tunnel. I love this stuff. I'm on my fifth bottle and when one bottle is half full then I buy another one."

-- **Sharrell A Brown, March 25, 2014**

"I found this on **thelovevitamin.com** and decided to try it. I have had cystic acne for years and have tried everything from cleansing to pharmaceuticals (including three rounds of Accutane). I noticed a difference after two weeks, and within a month I was only breaking out half as much. It took three months for my acne to disappear completely, but I have to take it three times a day. When I took it twice a day I still had breakouts right before my period. I have been taking it for six months and I don't know if I will ever be able to go without it as some users have been able to. I recommend this to all of my friends with the same problem! It's a miracle in a bottle!"

-- **L. Stone, March 18, 2014**

Reviews from Makeup Alley Blog

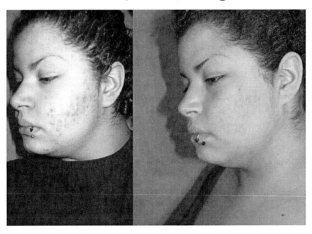

"I'm 37. I started to get really reallllly bad acne mostly along my jawline a couple of months after stopping Orthro Tricyclen. While I was on the pill, my skin was perfect. I got off because I didn't want to be taking hormones anymore. I tried soooo many things. None of them made my acne manageable. Estro Block® freaking worked. I bought the regular strength and started with three a day. I was almost completely clear after two weeks. I did eventually step it up to the pro strength, which is what I take now. I take three a day and plan to drop down to two and then one eventually. I don't have any more acne."

-- Olive, February 3, 2014

"I'm surprised there isn't a review of Estro Block® yet! In my mid-thirties I all of a sudden started developing painful, large, cystic acne along my jawline and on my upper neck. Usually two to three cysts at one given time, and then an additional two cysts during my period. They were deep seated and lasted for a very long, long time, also leaving a dark mark after disappearing. The cysts were very painful. I didn't see a doctor because I knew they'd put me on Retin-A or birth control. I knew the problem was internal. I could write a list of every scrub, cream, organic soap, and home-remedy, cleanse, etc. that I tried to get rid of the cysts. I have probably spent thousands of dollars looking for "the cure." I started taking Estro Block® (ordered from Amazon) approximately one and one-half months ago, and since then, I have had only two pimples emerge and they disappeared within three days. I take two capsules a day. I also have cleaned up my diet by eating less sugar and drinking less alcohol as well eating more fruits and vegetables. However, I don't worry any more about getting cysts. I plan on continuing to use it and may try stopping periodically to see if I really need it anymore. If the cysts start coming back, then I plan to simply re-purchase a bottle. Please message me if you have any questions about it. I'm not a doctor, so it may be in your best interest to ask a doctor before starting any type of supplement."

-- Sara Mason, November 26, 2013

One last story: I had a young lady come into our office in Costa Mesa, California, in February 2014, after she had achieved remarkable results clearing up acne cysts using Estro Block® for four months. She asked me why her dermatologist wasn't aware of Estro Block®. I told her I would supply scientific papers showing how and why this approach can improve one's skin.

We believe this book about natural methods will help educate everyone about acne and healthier skin. I trust you will be as successful as many thousands of our participants and readers.

Please go to our website estroblock.com for continuation of the story of estrogen dominance and its related symptoms.

Appendix 3

QUESTIONS AND ANSWERS FOR ACNE

Birth Control Pills

Q Is Estroblock safe to use while using birth control pills?

A. Yes, not only is Estro Block® safe to use during the use of birth control pills, it may be one of the best ways to protect one from the potential and dangerous side effects of the "Synthetic Pill" because Estro Block® clears these dangerous bad estrogens while restoring the good estrogens. I would also, if I were you, consider the use of the Liv D Tox™ as it will work synergistically with Estro Block® to clear other forms of harmful metabolites of estrone. There is actual more synthetic estrone (the bad estrogen) in synthetic hormones. The benefit of Estro Block® is that it may reduce some of the symptoms or problems created by birth control pills.

Pregnancy

Q. Is Estro Block® safe to take while trying to conceive? A. Yes Estro Block® or Estro Block Pro®, and Liv DTox™ are all safe because they contain GRAS (generally regarded as safe) ingredients. Take no more than one capsule a day. The safety of cruciferous vegetables while trying to conceive has been verified by animal studies where animals given high dosages of cruciferous phytochemicals have successfully reproduced.

Under ideal conditions, when a women plans to become pregnant, she must be following a healthy whole unprocessed foods diet including yams, avocados, vegetables, beans, peas, brown rice, and fruit with sufficient calories to be at her ideal body weight.

Nursing

Q. Can I nurse my baby while taking Estro Block®?

A. Yes. Stay within the suggested dosages of a person under 150 lbs.; that is two capsules taking one in the morning and one in the afternoon or evening with a meal. Many women have checked with their doctors and they felt Estro Block® or Estro Block Pro would be safe during pregnancy or nursing using the lower dosages of one or two a day.

Q. What additional supplements can I take while pregnant?

A. RAD Iodine can be taken every other day to get the necessary Iodine supporting healthy brain development in children. We also recommend you use Stay Young (which is rich in B12, Folic Acid and B3), take Pro Vitamin D3, and get your omega EPA/DHA from marine algae.

Young Male Hormone Balance

Q. Are young boys affected by acne from estrogen imbalances?

A. Yes, young boys are now developing acne, breast enlargement, or obesity due to estrogen dominance. Young men lose their ability to mature into healthy, virile men. Have your boys eat healthy foods, exercise, and take Estro Block® at suggested amounts for those under 180 lbs.

Success in Clearing Acne balancing hormones

Q. Can elevated levels of androgens, particularly DHT and androstenedione, cause hirsutism (abnormal hair growth in women), alopecia (hair loss) and acne?

A. Although it is true that elevated androgen levels will increase symptoms such as acne, the drug approach will cause side effects. The more natural solution to acne, with your doctor's permission, is to get the cause of the problem. The Delgado Protocol teaches that hormones work in certain balances. Catabolic must balance with anabolic, and the adrenals and cortisol levels are affected by androgens, which is influenced by estrogen levels.

Q. Do you have any success stories of people improving their acne or skin with Estro Block®?

A. See Tracy's story on The Love Vitamin **http://www.thelovevitamin.com**, and bloggers such as Fran Kerr **Highonclearskin.com** and several others with excellent results. These people are not paid by us and discovered Estro Block® by word of mouth. See **Estroblock.com** for more actual stories. You can also visit Instagram.

How Long Should I Wait Before I See Results In Reducing Acne?

Q: I've been using this for over a month and I have not seen any changes to my hormonal acne.

A. Your hormonal levels depend on the amount of toxins in your body, the foods you eat, your body weight, and your daily exercise habits. Although some people see results as quickly as one or two months it can take as long as six months to properly balance the hormones. It is perfectly safe to increase or even double your capsule servings to see quicker results.

Q. Why is my urine orange?

A. You may notice as Estro Block® detoxifies your body, the color of your urine may temporarily change to an orange/brown color. This is normal and is a good sign the product is working. Some people who have stopped taking Estro Block® and then resumed, notice the dark color in the urine returns until your body finishes phase 1 of detoxification.

If you are concerned about orange urine, consider increasing your hydration to at least eight glasses a day and reducing your meat/dairy intake. Also Adrenal DMG, LivDTox, Stay Young and Slim Blend Protein will assist in the release and cleansing.

Estro Block is like eating two lbs. of raw cruciferous vegetables a day and Estro Block Pro is like consuming four lbs. of raw cruciferous vegetables a day. Support the use of this product by improving your food selection to include more raw vegetables such as baby bok choy, Napa cabbage, Brussel sprouts and broccoli in your diet.

Strong Smell of Estro Block® Is Good

Q: Estro Block® has a very strange potent smell if I open up a capsule. Is that normal?

A: That is the natural smell (almost like "moth balls") of a high grade indole-3-carbinol-I3C and Diindolylmethane DIM from cruciferous vegetables such as cabbage, Brussels sprouts, broccoli, cauliflower, and kale. This smell is normal. The stronger the smell, the more effective the product. Other products have far less potency because they are masked in blends (like broccoli powder) and filler ingredients that offer little or no benefit. Our products are free of fillers, excipients, stearates, and other artificial ingredients that sometimes mask these natural scents.

ACNE from PCOS

Q: I have been told I have acne because of PCOS. What will help with polycystic ovary syndrome (PCOS)?

A. Studies show that people with PCOS tend to have high androgens, specifically high DHEA and high androstenedione. This converts either into the bad estrogens and/or converts into DHT and testosterone on the skin as the chart illustrates in appendix.

Once your hormone levels have been properly evaluated you many need a combination of Estro Block®, Liv DtoxTM, estriol cream and progesterone cream. Some may benefit with a prescription of BiEst (Estradiol and Estriol in a cream) from an anti-aging doctor.

Also, a change in diet towards mostly plant based meals will inhibit PCOS. Studies show that in cultures (like those in Papua New Guinea, Africa and parts of Asia) consuming diets low in fat and high in plant foods have almost no instances of acne, PCOS, etc.

Thyroid Health

Q: Will the cruciferous vegetables in Estro Block® affect my thyroid?

A. Dr. Joel Furhman at his web site drfuhrman.com does an excellent job explaining the safety of cruciferous vegetables as it relates to thyroid function and says there is no harm caused to the thyroid function. Estro Block® provides benefits without affecting thyroid.

However, there are areas of the USA and in the world where Iodine is in poor supply. Then RAD Iodine can help support healthy levels and help the skin. Occasionally we have some people who have thyroid imbalances so severe they need a natural bio identical thyroid T3 and T4 from compound pharmacy with a prescription or to use a whole thyroid glandular.

Estrogen Levels: Good or Bad

Q: I have heard there is a shift of estrogen levels from a bad form to a good form after the consumption of Estro Block®, is that true?

A. There is a beneficial increase in a good form of estrogen called two-hydroxestrone (2OHE) with a decrease in a dominate form called 16aOHE because Estro Block® or Estro Block Pro® provide Cytochrome P450 Enzymes to metabolize or reduce toxic forms of "bad" estrogen. Estro Block® insures protective factors, and allows the body to function at its best. As your hormones are regulated your skin and health can improve.

Q: My gynecologist thinks I might be starting pre-menopause. Can I still take Estro Block®?

A. For pre-menopause women, if your levels are proven low by hormone testing and your estriol is considerably lower than estrone and estradiol, then you may notice benefits from the use of progesterone cream and estriol cream in conjunction with Estro Block®. Using Estro Block® will insure that most of the restoration of estrogen balance will come from the good forms of estrogens (2OHE as measured in the urine), than the bad forms of estrogen (16aOHE).

Stopping Estrogen Dominance Improves your overall health

Q. What results have been reported using the ingredients in Liv DTox™ with Estro Block® and a healthier diet?

A. The ingredients of Liv DTox™ are highly supportive of a healthier immune system. Men (under their doctor's guidance) appear to show reduced PSA levels when combined with daily use of pomegranate juice and a diet rich in fiber and mostly unprocessed foods. The Delgado Protocol is now in main stream medical journals by Dean Ornish and the work of the Pritikin researchers I worked with years ago. Women have reported fibroid, cyst or tumor reduction when combining the ingredients of LivDTox™ with a mostly vegan, raw, unprocessed food diet free of sugar, separated fats, meats, or dairy.

Q. What other issues may also resolved besides acne using Estro Block®, Liv DTox™, TestroVida™, Adrenal DMG™, Progesterone cream, Stay Young™ in conjunction with your Simply Healthy diet and Delgado Protocol for Health™ plan?

A. Users of the above program have found resolution or improvement of the following: Polycystic ovary syndrome (PCOS), infertility, ovarian cysts, mid-cycle pain, puffiness and bloating, cervical dysplasia (abnormal pap smear), rapid weight gain, breast tenderness, mood swings, heavy bleeding, anxiety, depression, migraine headaches, insomnia, foggy thinking, red flush on face, gallbladder problems, and weepiness. Estrogen excess leads to building more lining within the endometrium (uterus lining) leading to excess bleeding, which leads to millions of unnecessary hysterectomies.

When will Experts on Acne agree?

Q. Why are many doctors, dermatologists, and bloggers unaware of your discovery that acne is principally caused by hormonal and estrogen imbalances?

A. I believe this natural approach has been missed because so much attention and advertising is focused on medications like Accutane, antibiotics, synthetic hormones, Proactiv, benzoyl peroxide therapy used off label. This new approach is gaining rapid acceptance with each success.

Q: What if I was told my acne problem is genetic?

A. When identical twins are compared to fraternal twins we see an 80% correlation to genetic factors related to acne. However these genetic tendencies can be overcome with a total approach to skin care starting with the internal hormones.

Q. Why is Estro Block Pro®, Triple strength your best-selling product?

A. Estro Block Pro® not only contains the largest amount of DIM on the market per capsule, it also has wasabi root which is 40x higher in isothiocyanates than broccoli and other important ingredients that may detoxify one's body and colon at the deepest level. This product is free of gluten, soy, or additives and made in the USA in a GMP pharmaceutical certified laboratory.

Can I Get A Cheaper Brand?

Q: Aren't there cheaper high-quality estrogen blockers at natural food grocers that will have the same results?

A. There may be some Estro Block® mimics. Often, to reduce costs, they hide the most important ingredients into what is called a "blend." Beware that in the long run you are paying far more money without getting the deep level of cleansing necessary. The competitors that we have analyzed in the less than $25 category have ONLY 12 mg of DIM because their blend lists 100 mg including other fillers and ingredients.

Estro Block® Regular I3C has significantly more DIM and other active ingredients for only $9 more per bottle. Also the added ingredient I3C is in the perfect ratio to DIM in a proprietary combinations. Look at the comparison charts in the Appendix section.

Diet, Raw Food, Fiber, Insulin

Q. Can elevated insulin levels cause acne? And which foods are the worst for my insulin control?

A. Yes. The worst foods that increase insulin levels and acne are cow's milk, cheese, eggs, butter, oils of all types, and meat of all types including chicken, fish, and pork. Even a fake food vegetarian plant-based diet that includes sugar and oils or high fat tofu and excess processed foods can promote acne as it can alter hormonal balances of estrogen, which increase in the gut in the presence of excess separated fats or oils). However a clean vegan diet, rich in fiber intake including walnuts, beans, peas, yams, fruit and vegetables will do wonders for your insulin levels and your skin.

Q. What foods are a good source of protein, yet still improve my hormone levels?

A. The foods best known as sources of proteins for humans (not relying on outdated rat studies) that can be absorbed without harming insulin or hormonal balance are: yams, purple sweet potatoes, sweet potatoes of all varieties, golden Yukon potatoes, beets, squash, asparagus, soaked nuts, soaked seeds, chia seeds, peas, brown rice, lentils, beans, all vegetables, most fruit, and small amounts of whole sources of fat such as coconut and avocado.

The vegetable foods that will improve hormonal balance to help prevent estrogen dominance and acne are those rich in

DIM and other important phytochemicals in foods prepared raw or steamed with less water. Sources of DIM per half cup: Brussels sprouts 104 mg, garden cress, mustard greens, turnips, savoy cabbage, kale, watercress, kohlrabi, red cabbage, broccoli, horseradish, cauliflower, and bok choy 19 mg.

Q. Will my gut health affect my skin?

A. Yes, eat sauerkraut, dairy free yogurt from coconut, and Korean Kim Chee, along with probiotics. We use a product called Slim Blend Protein which is also rich in probiotics, fiber, organic, with over 30 whole foods kept at under 118 degrees to preserve the enzymes.

Medications to Control Acne

Q. Should I take prescription medications to suppress DHT such as Spiro lactone or fine astride for acne?

A. Our theory is that reducing harmful forms of estrogen will allow testosterone to be restored to a better ratio of three parts to one part DHT, thereby getting to the cause of the problem. Ask your doctor if you can give this herbal phytochemical and healthy lifestyle approach a chance for 6 months, and you can always revisit the medications.

Antibiotics, Corticosteroids & Acne

Q. Will antibiotics be my best course of therapy for acne?

A. The reason the research overwhelmingly warns against the use of antibiotics and medications is not because they don't work, (as many have experienced, they can work very well) but because both have potentially problematic long term side effects. Our bodies have more bacteria than we have human cells. The antibiotics destroy the good along with elevated levels of bad bacteria. A healthy gut depends on bacteria for several functions including improve our immune system. What's more, their use represents the exact opposite approach to healing we practice in the field of integrative health. Regular use of Antibiotics can impede your body's natural defenses.

Q. Can medications such as Lithium, isoniazid, diphenylhydantoin cause acne?

A. Yes, several medications can cause acne. Check with your doctor to use our protocol.

Q. Will Retin A help my skin?

A. Initially Retin A may help, however it can be harsh on your skin and liver (while doing nothing for your hormonal balance).

The approach of the integrative health and anti-aging community is one that promotes detoxifying the liver and boosting your natural immunity. EstroBlock works by clearing away the xenoestrogens that damage hormonal metabolism in the body.

It is part of a lifestyle choice to also avoid toxins, pesticides, chemical ridden cosmetics, GMO food, fatty over processed meats and dairy.

Stress, Liver Detox & Acne

Q. Will corticosteroids like prednisone cure my acne?

A. IF you are under stress, try using Adrenal DMG™, a natural way to support the adrenal glands without the risk of prednisone. William McKinnley Jeffries MD in his book *Safe uses of Cortisol* explains how the adrenals are supported by natural cortisol and herbs. Adrenal DMG can have a positive impact on your adrenal function, energy and immune system. Herbs in this product detoxify the liver and help with energy and most natural chemical reactions of the liver. Some natural herbal ingredients target RNA and DNA viruses, and bacteria. Caprylic Acid fights fungus (candida). Take up to six to eight a day for relief.

We also find the skin improves when you support liver function with DMG, an ingredient in this product proven to enhance over 500 natural biochemical reactions in the liver.

Q. Why do you suggest the use of Adrenal DMG™ for acne clients?

A. Adrenal DMG offers methylation from dimethylglycine to assist the liver in several important biochemical reactions the body must undergo every day. There is a need for adrenal support to help fight acne related stress. Adrenal Cortex, and certain herbs improve the immune system and are critical to overall good health to establish beauty from within.

Q. What if I have the flu or a cold? Can I take Estro Block®?

A. If you have cold or flu-like symptoms, it may be a sign you have low adrenal function and are unable to produce enough cortisol to fight the stress of illness. Get your adrenal function tested by a saliva or urine test for cortisol. When you're improving the ratio of hormones, if the anabolic levels increase above the catabolic levels, Estro Block® will not solve the adrenal deficiency.

The solution is to support your adrenals with Adrenal DMG™ along with the use of Liv DTox™, and get additional daylight exposure on your skin to stimulate improved adrenal function. You also might notice improvement in your energy.

Q: I just purchased some 175 mg Milk Thistle to take with the Estro Block®· Why exactly is this recommended?

A: Some people recommend Milk Thistle to help the liver through the detox process. This is not necessary for everyone but it may help.

Support Supplements to reduce Acne

Q. I have a stubborn case of acne. Can I take higher dosages and liver support supplements?

A. Some people may break out if their liver is functioning below normal. Correction in estrogen hormones can increase the need of the liver to process out chemicals and hormones. Use Estro Block® in combination with Liv DTox™.

If you are under 180 lbs take initially three capsules per day spaced four hours apart. If you are over 180 lbs., take six capsules (2 capsules every four hours). Look to do this program for a minimum of three months before lowering the amount.

Q. Are there side effects from taking too much EstroBlock of Liv DTox?

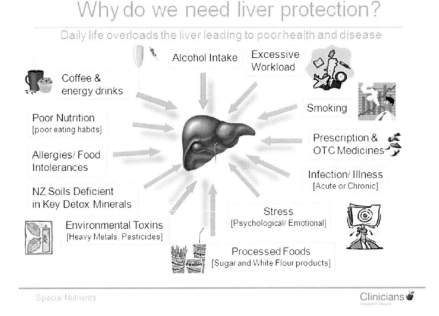

Why do we need liver protection?

Daily life overloads the liver leading to poor health and disease

Coffee & energy drinks

Poor Nutrition
[poor eating habits]

Allergies/ Food Intolerances

NZ Soils Deficient in Key Detox Minerals

Environmental Toxins
[Heavy Metals, Pesticides]

Alcohol Intake

Excessive Workload

Smoking

Prescription & OTC Medicines

Infection/ Illness
[Acute or Chronic]

Stress
[Psychological/ Emotional]

Processed Foods
[Sugar and White Flour products]

Special Nutrients

Clinicians

A. Any side effects from EstroBlock and LivDtox are typically short term and are generally related to the detoxifying process. These effects can be mitigated by adjusting dosages and through some other methods mentioned in this book or at our website EstroBlock.com.

Adrenal DMG is also a potent methylator which assists the liver in processing over 20 different chemical reactions.

Q. What will Stay Young™ provide me in my fight against acne?

A. Stay Young™ has the necessary full B12 and folic acid spectrum for healthy skin. Stay Young™ also supports healthy nitric oxide levels to help counter oxidation and free radical damage. Free radical damage leads to aging of the skin and can worsen acne. Stay Young™ also supports healthy chromosome replication which improves the length of the telomeres to slow the aging process.

Q. Will zinc and vitamin D3 help my acne?

A. Yes, if your levels are low, then supplements with Zinc and Vitamin D3 with probiotics will help.

Q. Can TestroVida Pro™ be used if I have acne?

A. Yes, after about six months, when you have stabilized your estrogen levels with Estro Block® or Estro Block Pro®, and if you are taking Adrenal DMG™ and or Liv DTox™, then experiment with adding TestroVida Pro™, as it is generally excess DHT levels rather than testosterone that causes acne. TestroVida Pro™ has no testosterone in it, nor DHEA as other so called testosterone boosters. This all natural herbal approach will allow your hormone levels to reach youthful levels without becoming excessive. That way you can enhance your libido and firm up your body while maintaining healthy skin.

Q: Can I just take DHEA instead of Estro Block®?

A. DHEA in oral form, typically taken in amounts of 20-50 mg. has been known to cause acne. Ray Sahelian, MD, states that amounts exceeding five mg orally should be avoided. Additional evidence shows that DHEA tends to be effective in the form of acne that appears in patients that have autoimmune conditions such as lupus. In this case, it is also necessary to take Vitamin B5 (pantothenic acid), which can be helpful in reducing acne. Research indicates that taking DHEA in transdermal or cream form is safe in doses up to 10 mg per day with less likelihood to convert into other hormones that tend to aggravate or cause acne.

Clean Skin, Dirt & Acne

Q. Does dirt cause acne?

A. No, dirt is not associated with acne. Office workers have just as much acne compared to construction workers exposed to a lot of dirt and grime. Beauty starts from within, and your skin is the organ that releases toxins and protects you from harmful bacteria or dirt. Washing with chemical-free bath items may improve your skin condition. Some people rinse their face with filtered purified water and have noticed some improvement in their skin over using harsh tap water and soaps. There is an interesting movement called the caveman regimen, which follows some of the suggestions from Tracey of the Love Vitamin. They choose not to wash their face for 30 days to prove that some of these harsh chemicals are actually contributing to acne.

Q. Will rubbing or friction cause acne?

A. Yes. Bra straps, backpacks, and chin straps can cause inflammation at the site of the hair follicles, and, with sweating or pressure, can cause acne.

Suggested Serving Size & Use of Estro Block®

Q. How many capsules of regular Estro Block® or Estro Block Pro, triple strength can I take per day beyond what the label says?

A. To improve your odds against acne or restore balance to the hormonal cascade use Estro Block regular if you are less than 150 lbs. If you are over 150 lbs. you can use Estro Block Pro®. The capsule amount will vary from person to person depending on the severity of your acne. Those with mild cases may benefit from as few as two capsules a day. It is fine to increase your dosage to 3 or 4 capsules a day, each capsule spaced about three or four hours apart until you see results. Then reduce the capsule amount to maintenance levels of one capsule per day to sustain your healthy looking skin once you see significant improvement.

Q. Does Estro Block® always have to be taken with a meal?

A. Estro Block® should be taken with a nutrient rich meal however it is still effective when taken on an empty stomach.

Side Effects & Solutions

Q: I suffer from pretty severe headaches in general but noticed that since taking the Estro Block® my headaches have gotten worse. Is this a side effect that others have suffered from?

A. Headaches can come from estrogen dominance while having low progesterone levels in women. In addition to Estro Block you may need progesterone cream. Drink plenty of water and hydrate. Sometimes the detoxification process needs to progress slower in sensitive individuals (causing headaches) so reduce dosage to one capsule a day for one week then increase adding a second capsule later in the day.

Q: What if Estro Block® makes me break out?

A: It is a rare occurrence for people to break out using Estro Block®, but if they do (or are concerned about it), they should take some added steps. Hormonal acne responds best to improvements in the diet along with supplements. Eat more foods like rich cruciferous vegetables to improve hormonal balance. We also suggest following a Simply Healthy diet low in oils, meats, and dairy and rich in whole foods.

Q. Can I take Estro Block Pro® and Liv Dtox™ if I'm already under treatment with Tamoxifen for cancer?

A. Yes, many doctors have encouraged there patient to add natural phytochemical ingredients as found in Estro Block® or Estro Block Pro® with Liv Dtox™ (cell Stabilizer).

Doctor's awareness of your protocol's for acne

Q. Are Anti-Aging doctors who specialize in hormonal balance seeing the benefits in treating acne by protocols like yours?

A. Other doctors, including Jonathan Wright, MD, as interviewed in the book *I'm Too Young for This* by Suzanne Somers, Ron Rothenberg, UC San Diego Professor, Thierry Hertoghe, MD, Sangeeti Pati, MD, and Naina Sachdev, MD, have observed the connection of estrogen dominance to acne.

We realized that DHT becomes more potent in the skin as the body attempts to compensate for excessive estrogen as measured in urinary metabolites. This is why products like Estro Block® and the additional support protocol of supplements with a healthier diet and exercise can help clear up your skin.

Q. What Should I Tell My Doctor About Estro Block®?

A. Encourage your doctor to find out about this all-natural approach to clearing up the acne and other related disorders associated with hormonal imbalances by having your doctor call us or visit our web site at **www.Estroblock.com**.

Estro Block® Hormonal Connection to Acne

Q. My doctor, a dermatologist, has never heard of this estrogen hormonal connection to acne. What is the technical answer he or she will understand?

A. Estro Block® and LivDTox™ improve liver enzyme interactions; the modification of estrogen metabolites also produces an ultimate state in which more of the 2-hydroxyestrogens relative to 16a-hydroxyestrogens and 4-hydroxyestrogens results in less overall estrogenic actions in vivo. This is due to induction (activation) of the estradiol-2-hydroxylase enzyme, an enzyme that converts estrogens and estrone to their 2-hydroxylated form which is seen as chemo protective and in some cases anti-estrogenic. This then allows healthy ratios of estrogen, sex hormone binding globulin and improved levels of androgens. Specifically the DHT reduces, no longer having to compete with high levels of unmetabolized estrone or estradiol.

Q. Why do doctors often ignore estrogen and think it is best to suppress androgen levels with synthetic hormones or medications?

A. The original theories about the cause of acne were based on the assumption that the androgen hormones were the only cause of acne. However, I have observed the complex interaction of estrogen and its effect on androgen. Doctors wanted to suppress the androgens without knowing the origin of acne. We now know there is a complex balance of hormones influenced by phytochemicals, diet, and lifestyle, solving the mystery of acne. Many people like the idea of getting to the cause of the problem rather than covering up the symptoms.

Lab Tests to detect the causes of acne

Q. What tests in saliva or blood hormones will detect the risk of acne?

A. High level of androstenedione, high free testosterone, and excess levels of DHEA, excess Estradiol, or excess estrone in saliva or blood all have been found to cause acne. We find the 24-hour urine test for hormones to be the most accurate in detecting harmful estrogens (16aOHE) and their effect on androgens which leads to acne. We offer this test, yet most doctors rarely utilize it because they haven't been trained to do urine tests, depending mostly on blood tests. The goal is to achieve balance, not too high or too low, and a proper ratio of each of the hormones working together.

Q. Will these saliva, blood or urine lab tests always be the most sensitive way to guide me to improve my skin and health?

A. No, your lab tests may be "normal" and you may still have acne. There are more sophisticated tests that can measure enzyme activity in the skin, which increases the conversion of hormone metabolites such as DHT, androstenedione, Free

Testosterone, or Estrone in the skin. These types of tests are only done in research labs.

Q. What other lab tests are needed to monitor to reduce acne?

A. The tests in the blood for SHBG (high levels of SHBG tend to reduce acne), insulin (high levels increases risk of acne), luteinizing hormone LH, glucose and lipids which include triglycerides (high levels of fat in the blood cause the insulin to become desensitized, which will increase the risk of diabetes, lupus, and acne).

Appendix 4

ACNE SOLUTIONS & NUTRIENT SUPPORT

Note: Nutrients may be repeated because they support several bodily functions. These statements related to health claims or expectations have not been evaluated by the Food and Drug Administration. This product is not intended to diagnose, treat, cure or prevent any disease.

Hormone Imbalances

Nutrient	Ideal Daily Amount	Suggested Products
Diindolylmethane (DIM)	100 to 900 mg	Estro Block®
Indole-3-carbinol (I3C)	40 to 240 mg	
Wasabi Root	40 to 200 mg	Estro Block Pro®
D-Glucoruonolactone	100 to 200 mg	
Chrysin	50 to 200 mg	
DHEA	5 mg to 10 mg	Testro Vida Cream

Broccoli extract	100 to 500 mg	DHT Block
Watercress extract	50 to 100 mg	
Cabbage extract	25 to 100 mg	
Adrenal Extract	30 to 60 mg	Adrenal DMG™
Natural phyto-chemicals in cream		Estro Block Cream available soon
Progesterone, Estradiol, Estriol		EstroBlock Cream
Estriol		Estriol Cream
Growth factors		Grow Young™
Amino Acids Growth Factor		Renuva

Liver Detoxification (Cleanse)

Nutrient	Ideal Daily Dose	Suggested Products
Astragalus Root (10 to 1) Tumeric Root	250 to 750 mg	Liv DTox™ contains all of these ingredients to help cleanse the face and body, assisting the liver to remove toxins and excess estrogen
Cyperus Root Asparagus Root Pomegranate Fruit	100 to 400 mg	
Ginger Root	20 to 100 mg	
Milk Thistle-Silymarin	20 to 200 mg	

Skin & cell repair by Methylation support DNA

Nutrient	Ideal Daily Amount	Suggested Products
		Stay Young™

		PM:
Acetyl-L-Carnitine Blend:	760 to 1500 mg	Contains in blend
Vitamin B12		
Methylcobalamin		
Cyanocobalamin		
Vitamin B1		
Folic Acid-5MTHF		Stay Young AM
CoQ10		
RNA, DNA		
Blueberry Fruit		
Alpha Lipoic Acid		
S-adenosylmethionine (SAMe)		Doctors Best
methylsulfonylmethane (MSM)		Renuva
betaine from betaine hydrochloride		
5-methyltetrahydrofolate		Stay Young AM

Digestive cleansing for healthy skin

Nutrient	Ideal Daily Amount	Suggested Products
Flax seed Golden	30 grams blend	Slim Blend Protein™
Seed sprouts, organic		All these ingredients are contained in Slim Blend Pro
Chia, Millet, Amaranth		

Brown Rice Protein		
Vegetable, organic		
Beet, Carrot, Parsley		
Fruit blend		
Probiotics, Enzymes, Vitamins, Minerals		Slim Blend Pro

Inflammation reducers, immune system enhance

Nutrient	Ideal Daily Amount	Suggested Products
Ashwagandha DMG- Dimethylglycine	Blend 600 to 1200 mg	Adrenal DMG™ contains all in blend
Echinacea Purpurea		
Black Cherry Root		
Cranberry		
Lomatium dissectum		
Caprylic Acid		
Adrenal cortex Policosanol Garlic bulb Grape Fruit Seed		
Mushroom, organic	Blend 10 grams	Stem Cell Strong™ Contains all in blend
Algae Blend		

MACA, MSM,		
Long Jack		
Tart Cherry		
Resveratrol		
American Ginseng		
Ginkgo Biloba		
Pumpkin Seed		Stem Cell Strong

Reducers of Fats, Lipids, Sugar, insulin

Nutrient	Ideal Daily Amount	Suggested Products
Irvingia Gabonensis	Blend 790 mg	Lean N Fit™ These ingredients are in formula
Caralluma Fimbrata		
Kudzu root		
Paullinia Cupana		

Oxidative stress, free radical scavengers, circulation, supports healthy cell formation

Nutrient	Ideal Daily Amount	Suggested Products
Nitric Oxide support:	700 to 1,400 mg	Stay Young PM™ capsules
Beet Root		
L-Citruline		
Kale leaf	770 to 1,500 mg	Stay Young™ AM Chewable- ingredients support

		healthy cells
Red Spinach Leaf		Stay Young AM
Hawthorn Berry		
Pomegranate		
L-Carnosine		
Long Jack fruit	200 to 1	TestroVida Pro
Oat Straw Avena Sativa		
Muira Puama		
Nettle Leaf		
Hemp CBD		Immune Strong
Green Tea Leaf Extract & Blueberry Fruit		
Acetyl-L-Carnosine		
Alpha Lipoic Acid		
CO-Enzyme Q10		
Quebracho Blanco		
DNA, RNA		Lean N Fit
Astragalus Root (10 to 1)	250 to 750 mg	Liv DTox™ / Cell Stabilizer
Tumeric Root	200 to 600 mg	
Cyperus Root	100 to 400 mg	
Asparagus Root	100 to 300 mg	
Pomegranate Fruit	75 to 500 mg	
Silymarin, Milk Thistle	20 to 300 mg	
Ginger Root	20 to 80 mg	

EstroBlock

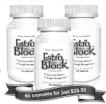

COMPARISON TO OTHER DIM PRODUCTS

Compare the Products. Draw your own Conclusion

The following are comparisons of EstroBlock® to other well known, competing products on the consumer market. They all claim to produce similar results, but we invite you to see for yourself how they really match when compared side by side with Estro Block®.

60 capsules for just $29.99

Expensive? Not Really. Here's Why.

We've created this handy chart to help savvy consumers like you see past all the hype. At first glance, some of these products seem like they might be a good bargain...but look again. Upon further inspection, they don't seem to be such good bargains after all.

Try Estro Block® Regular or Pro. There's an Estro Block® for everyone!

In each capsule of Estro Block® there is a powerful balancing blend of DIM and 13C for reducing fat-bulding estrogens and restoring good estrogens, combined with high concentrations of Ciindolylmethane to rinse clean your inner body. We use a special process that allows the DIM in Estro Block® to become 5 times more effective than crystalline DIM, so two capsules equal over two pounds of raw cruciferous vegetables. You can take Estro Block® every day and night to correct imbalances of estrogens. Adjust your dosage if needed.

DIM Bio Response

Contains only 25 mg of DIM and retails for $11.99 at just 25% the amount of DIM in Estro Block®. One would have to purchase 4 DIM Bio Response bottles in order to receive the same amount given in just one bottle of Estro Block®. $48.00 versus $29.00? That's quite a difference.

EstroBalance

Has (at most) 35 mg of DIM per tablet. Even with 60 tablets you would have to buy 3 bottles at $40.00 each (which equals $120.00) to match what is in regular Estro Block® for $29.00. This comes out to an additional spending of $100.00.

Estrosense

Estrosense offers 150 mg of Indole 3 Carbinol per 2 capsules (75 mg for one) and 50 mg of DIM for 2 capsules (25 mg for one). It is highly overpriced at $22.00. One would have to order 2 bottles of Estrosense to match just one bottle of Estro Block Pro®.

Royal Maca Plus for Women

Though it contains 100 mg of DIM per capsule, it contains less desirable "crystalline" type DIM and you would have to buy 5 bottles to come close to regular Estro Block®. Maca is a wonderful herb, but we recommend it in higher dosages than capsules can contain. Clinical dosages of Maca can be found in our scoopable food powder, called Stem Cell Strong.

Jarrow DIM+CDG

Contains 100 mg of DIM per capsule and costs $25.00 for a 30 count. That's closer to our Estro Block® but it is only a 30 count, not a 60 count. One would still have to buy 2 bottles to match the 60 capsules of regular Estro Block®, costing over $50.00. This will still come without the Wasabi and the Chrysin.

DIM-Plus

Contains 120 capsules for $33.00; however, the capsules only contain a tiny amount of DIM, 25 mg for 2 capsules! That means those taking DIM Plus are only getting 12 mg per capsule of DIM, and it includes...soy! Ultimately it would take 10 bottles of DIM Plus (330) to equal one bottle of the popular Estro Block®.

#1 Competitor With Estro Block

.

Appendix 5

WHY DO WE FEEL ESTRO BLOCK® IS BETTER THAN ITS COMPETITORS?

"Knockoffs" have no authorization to use the name Estro Block. They generally sell for a higher price with 50% less DIM than Estro Block Pro®. You get a few other ingredients that are not as potent and are improperly formulated.

The best advice for ideal results to improve your skin is to improve your diet with the cleanse plan listed in the appendix, take the supplements the match the most effective ways to balance your hormones based on the questionnaire in the appendix, and the lab test findings. Contact us for guidance if you have questions.

Estro Block® & Delgado Protocol Products Available Around the World

INTERNATIONAL:
Available soon In INDONESIA pending registration!

KLINIK GUNTUR INDONESIA

Products in Stock: Liv D'Tox, EB,
PNS, Adrenal DMG, Stay Young,
Protein Plus

Jl. Guntur No. 32 - Jakarta Selatan, Indonesia 12980
Phone: +62 21 828 0939 / +62 812 81 66 8852
Email: klinikguntur@gmail.com   Hours: 8.30 am to 5.30 pm

SUPER HEALTH AUSTRALIA

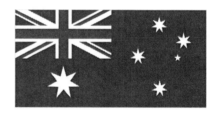

Products in Stock:
EB PRO, EB, Liv D'Tox

info@superhealth.com.ausuperhealth.com.au
Phone: 011419041554,

TOH SEK CHEONG (MALAYSIA)

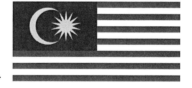

Products in Stock: Liv D'Tox, Ad-
renal DMG, EB PRO, Slim Blend PRO, LNF, PNS, Grow Young
Phone: 601-253-87311   sumrui@gmail.com

COHA HEALTH BERMUDA

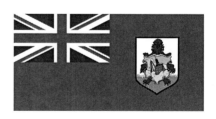

In Stock: Estro Block Pro, Testro
Vida, Stay Young, Adrenal DMG

78 Happy Valley Rd., Devonshire, DV03   Tel: 1-441-295-7612
Email: mail@cohahealth.com   Website: http://www.cohahealth.com/
For store hours visit our website as they vary.

PETE DAVANI LONDON

Products in Stock: EB PRO

peterdevani@gmail.com

Phone: 516-312-8833

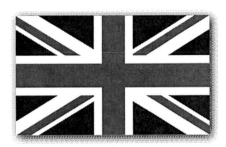

TBC MAY PING LI UK

Products in Stock: EB

mpli@live.com   Phone 61-
424922637

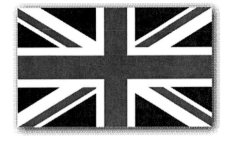

MIRIAM ZIELKE GERMANY

Products in Stock: EB PRO

info@carbundance.com   Phone: 01482213386

SAMUEL ASOMUGHA (SOUTH AFRICA)

Products in Stock: Adrenal DMG,
Testro Vida, RAD Iodine

drsamasomugha@yahoo.com234.803.307.9802

DR. LAUREN BRAMLEY & PARTNERS (HONG KONG)

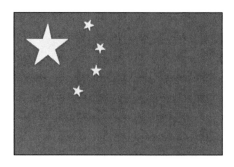

Products in Stock: Liv D'Tox

stefani@ibandp.com.hk

9/Floor, Pacific House, 20 Queens Road, Central, Hong Kong

Appendix 6

SUGGESTIONS TO CLEANSE YOUR SKIN BEYOND MEDICATIONS

Avoid chemicals & substances that harm skin

Offenders of the skin include alcohol, caffeine, and energy drinks such as Red Bull™, because they reduce the benefits of testosterone while increasing adverse effects on the skin, including oil formation and inflammation of sebum glands, thus causing acne.

Drugs prescribed off label: Not for their original intended use

As many medical experts will attest, drugs can offer great benefits in emergency or short-term applications, often off label, meaning other than its intended original use that causes undesirable side effects. Also longer term use of medications, including nutrient depletion can cause you serious harm.

One such example in the acne category is Accutane™ (a form of vitamin A). Warnings for Accutane™ include the risk of severe life- threatening birth effects, including birth defects of the ears, eyes, face, skull, heart and brain (**www.drugs.com**)

Accutane™ users are strongly advised to have regular liver enzyme screenings.

There are several medications prescribed for acne. Many of these medications do not offer a long term solutions. The drug prednisone also reduces the androgen production from the adrenal glands (*Safe Uses of Cortisol* by William McKinley Jeffries). This synthetic steroid therapy is harmful because there must be an equal balance between catabolic and anabolic hormones. When you interfere with this delicate balance of the adrenal hormones you may cause more colds, flu, and inflammatory pain in the body.

Another medication often used for acne is spirolactone. Spirolactone is used off label or longer than necessary it may suppress a necessary hormone in your body called aldosterone to prevent fluid retention. Yet holding fluids in your tissues is essential for good health.

Keep in mind your doctor is trying to help you and you can assist your doctor by employing these simple, yet effective methods to improve your skin and your overall health.

10-Day Express Cleanse Program

Day 1

Eliminate all:

Refined sugars-anything with added sucrose, high fructose corn syrup, or alcohol (cakes, cookies, candies, pastries, beer, wine, liquor)

Caffeinated drinks (sodas, coffee, tea)

Artificial colorings, flavorings, and sweeteners (packaged and processed foods)

Remove flesh foods (beef, pork, lamb, poultry, fish, wild game).

Eliminate Dairy (cheese, milk, yogurt, eggs)

Be sure to consume enough whole fresh food:

If you don't want to lose weight, then include extra whole foods: snacks with yams, sweet potatoes or jicama are better choices to sustain your energy. Enjoy large mixed salads, soups, or casseroles. You may wish to shorten and increase the intensity of your physical activities while snacking on Asian pears, watermelon, various fruit and vegetables during this ten day cleanse

Supplements:

Take one **scoop** of **Slim Blend Pro**™ mixed in a smoothie with healthy vegetables like bok choy, napa cabbage, carrots and fruits such as pears. Start with one **Estro Block**®, and **Adrenal DMG**™ capsule two times today, take one **Stay Young** capsule in the evening.

Day 2 & Day 3

In addition to eliminating foods listed for Days one, eliminate all:

Gluten grains – wheat, rye, barley, spelt, kamut, corn and oat

Note: You may continue to eat quinoa, rice, millet, and buckwheat

Continue with supplements same as day one and note improvements or responses.

Day 4-8

You have now eliminated all meat, fish, chicken, dairy, eggs, gluten or soy:

Use only grains (quinoa, rice, millet, buckwheat)

Have ¼ cup of Nuts and seeds (soak the nuts or seeds in water for three to eight hours to remove the anti-enzymes and bring to life the enzyme properties, just discard dark water, rinse and add to salads, smoothies or eat as snacks)

Note: You now should be eating large amounts (5 to 15 cups of vegetables, yams, and legumes with cruciferous vegetables (broccoli, cauliflower, kale, cabbage, Brussels sprouts)

Raw greens (red and green lettuce, romaine, spinach, endive)

Asparagus and green beans

Any fruit like fresh apples and pears (whole or freshly pureed in a smoothie)

Supplements:

Increase Slim Blend Pro™ by adding ½ scoop to 1 ½ total today

Take one Estro Block® capsule in the morning and one in the evening, with Adrenal DMG™ three capsules twice today. Take two capsules of Stay Young at night.

Day 8, 9

Avoid or reduce oils, olive oil, peanut oil, safflower oil, or butter, to less than ½ tsp per meal. Use lemon juice with spices or a fat free salad dressing like Warden Farm on your salads. Gradually continue to increase the amount of vegetables, squash, broccoli, lettuce, greens, and swiss chard to 15 to 20 cups a day. Have 3 to 5 servings of fruits a day, and use yams and beans for sufficient calories along with brown rice.

Day 10

Congratulations! You have successfully completed your 10-Day Express Program! For maximum benefit from this program, it is important to slowly reintroduce the foods to your diet one at a time. If you suspect that you have food allergies, try only one new food and wait 24-48 hours to see if you notice a reaction. If unsure about a reaction, wait until symptoms recede and eat only foods that do not cause a reaction. Then ingest the suspicious food again and take note. You can continue to make this healthy eating plan a way of life, with incredible amounts of nutrients, fiber.

Basic Dietary Guidelines for healthy skin and body:

Fruits Recommended: fresh, unsweetened, dried, frozen, water-packed fruits

Vegetables Recommended: all fresh raw, steamed, sautéed, juiced, or roasted vegetables

AVOID: corn; any creamed vegetables that have added sugar or milk

Complex unprocessed fiber, starches recommended: brown rice, oats, millet, quinoa, amaranth, tapioca, buckwheat, potatoes. AVOID: wheat, corn, all gluten-containing products

Breads & Cereals Recommended: Products made from brown rice, oat, buckwheat, millet, potato flour, tapioca, arrowroot, amaranth, or quinoa

AVOID: products made from wheat or containing yeast

Legumes Recommended: All legumes including peas and lentils (except soybeans)

AVOID: tofu, tempeh, soybeans, soy milk, and other soy products

Nuts & Seeds Recommended: almonds, cashews, pecans, walnuts, sesame (tahini), sunflower, pumpkin, nut butters (except peanut)

AVOID: peanuts, peanut butter

Dairy & Milk Substitutes Recommended: Almond Milk, Rice Milk, Coconut Milk, or other nut milks, egg replacer

AVOID: milk, cheese, cottage cheese, yogurt, butter, ice cream, frozen yogurt, non-dairy creamers, soy milk, and eggs

Fats: Recommended: avocado, flaxseed, safflower, sunflower, sesame, walnut, pumpkin, almond, grape seed

AVOID: processed and hydrogenated oils, margarine, butter, shortening, mayonnaise, spreads, poultry skin, deep fried foods, chips, donuts

Beverages: Recommended: filtered or distilled PH balanced water, decaffeinated herbal tea, seltzer or mineral water

AVOID: sodas, diet sodas, sports beverages, and other soft drinks and mixes; alcoholic beverages, coffee, tea, or other caffeinated beverages

Spices & Condiments: Recommended: vinegar (except malt); all spices including salt, pepper, cinnamon, cumin, dill, garlic, ginger, carob, oregano, parsley, dry mustard, rosemary, tarragon, thyme or turmeric

AVOID: chocolate, ketchup, chutney, soy sauce, BBQ sauce, bottled mustard, and other condiments

Sweeteners: Recommended: stevia, liquid or powder, Lo Hon GU, agave nectar, brown rice syrup, fruit sweeteners, blackstrap molasses

AVOID: white or brown refined sugar, honey, maple syrup, corn syrup, high fructose corn syrup, or evaporated cane sugar

AVOID THESE OTHER FOODS: processed foods containing baking soda or corn starch, processed starch foods containing any of the ingredients or sweeteners listed above.

Enjoy a variety of whole super foods daily. Start with a smoothie for breakfast or even a large salad that you continue to eat until lunch. We function best when we consume large amounts of fiber in whole foods. If you feel weak or hungry, snack on fresh food and fruit. Recipes from the *Simply Healthy* cookbook make excellent lunch and dinner options. The *Simply Healthy* cookbook provides the tastiest recipes based on the Delgado Diet that has been benefiting our clients for over 3 decades. We encourage you to consume more raw cruciferous vegetables (bok choy, Napa cabbage, broccoli, Brussel sprouts). We also promote eating more whole food, fiber rich yams, beans, vegetables, and brown rice. Asian (preferably Thai or Vietnamese) and Mediterranean-type diets (drop the olive oil, unless used on the skin) work best. Use meat, chicken, or fish only as flavoring in portions of less than 3 oz., three or four times a week.

A great source of balanced of hormones is herbal rich smoothies. We suggest adding the Slim Blend Pro, with over 30 super foods, probiotics, vitamins, minerals to provide a "complete meal." This special powder mix is prepared under the best conditions keeping the nutrients under 118 degrees to preserve all of the enzymes and phytochemicals normally destroyed by cooking.

Food Allergy Testing

Comprehensive 185 IgG Food Panel

Almond	Dill	Pepper, Black
Amaranth	Duck	Pepper, Chili

Anchovy
Apple
Apricot
Arrowroot
Artichoke
Asparagus
Avocado
Banana
Barley
Basil
Bass (Black)
Bay Leaf
Beah, Green
Bean, Lima
Bean, Pinto
Bean, Red
Beef
Beef, Red
Blackberry
Blueberry
Bran
Brazil Nut
Broccoli
Brussel Sprouts
Buckwheat
Buffalo
Cabbage
Canola
Cantaloupe
Capsicum
Carob
Carrot
Casein
Cashew
Cauliflower
Celery
Cheese, Bleu
Cheese, Cheddar
Cheese, Cottage
Cheese, Swiss
Cherry

Eggplant
Egg White
Egg Yolk
Fennel
Flaxseed
Flounder
Garlic
Ginger
Gingko Biloba
Ginseng
Gluten
Grape
Grapefruit
Haddock
Halibut
Hazelnut (Filbert)
Herring
Honey
Hops
Horseradish
Kiwi
Lamb
Lemon
Lentil
Lettuce
Licorice
Lime
Litchi
Lobster
Mackerel
Malt
Mango
Melon, Honeydew
Milk, Cow's
Milk, Goat's
Millet
Mushrooms
Mussel
Mustard
Navy Bean
Nutmeg

Pepper, Green
Pepper, Red
Peppermint
Perch, Sea
Pike, Walleye
Pineapple
Pistachio
Plum
Poppy Seed
Pork
Potato, Sweet
Potato, White
Pumpkin
Quinoa
Rabbit
Radish
Raspberry
Red Snapper
Rhubarb
Rice, Brown
Rosemary
Rye
Safflower
Sage
Salmon
Scallop
Sesame
Shrimp
Sole
Sorghum
Soybean
Spinach
Squash
Strawberry
Sugar Beet
Sugar, Cane
Sunflower
Swordfish
Tangerine
Tapioca
Tea, Black

Chestnut	Nutrasweet	Teff
Chicken	Oats	Thyme
Chick Pea (Garbanzo)	Okra	Tomato
Cinnamon	Olive, Green	Trout
Clam	Onion, White	Tuna
Cloves	Orange	Turkey
Cocoa	Oregano	Turmeric
Coconut	Oyster	Turnip
Codfish	Papaya	Vanilla Bean
Coffee	Paprika	Walnut, Black
Cola	Parsley	Watermelon
Corn	Parsnip	Wheat
Cottonseed	Pea, Black Eyed	Whey
Crab	Pea, Green	Whitefish
Cranberry	Peach	Yeast, Baker's
Cucumber	Peanut	Yeast, Brewer's
Date	Pear	Yogurt
Deer (Venison)	Pecan	Zucchini
	Pepper, Cayenne	

It is very important to have a personalized plan including foods best suited for you. The Alletess delayed food allergy blood testing for IgG is a good way to detect food incompatibilities. The test exposes 184 foods (listed above) to your own white blood cells and looks for signs of inflammation and rejection. If you have issues with sore joints, skin conditions, mood swings, aggression, depression or digestive problems then request a test kit. It will be sent to you with a requisition for your local lab.

We will get the results in four to five weeks and give you a copy to find out if you are compatible, mildly allergic, moderately allergic or severely allergic to 184 different foods, herbs, or spices including gluten, soy, dairy, meats, etc.

The IgG Alletess is a way to detect a problem food or allergen that otherwise cannot be detected by observing your reaction to the food. This is because an IgG reaction can cause symptoms over one week after consuming the offending food or herb.

When you get the color-coded test results, you can focus on consuming the foods and herbs that are "safe" for you. You can then eliminate or avoid the offending foods for at least 60 days. Then to test, gradually re-introduce the low offenders and to see if any symptoms return. Now you will have a way to further personalize your nutrition plan, instead of depending on less than accurate blood type, or skin patch testing for IGE, or muscle testing.

Supplements:

You must address supplementation because most people's diets are deficient even under the best conditions.

Be sure to take the supplements that provide B12-Methylcobalamin, 5-methyltetrahydrofolate (folic acid), Vitamin D3, probiotics and trace minerals.

Increase Slim Blend Pro™ by adding ½ scoop to 2 total today. This will give you sufficient protein, fiber, and organic nutrients as daily base to good health.

We find clients using Estro Block® (or Estro Block Pro® in more severe cases of acne or estrogen dominance or when an individual is greater than 15 lbs. overweight) are able to detoxify and metabolize more effectively. Metabolism is the safe breakdown of the harmful "bad" estrogens to a safer, healthier good estrogen.

Take one Estro Block® capsule in the morning and one in the evening. If you are more than 20 lbs. above your ideal weight, you may progress to EstroBlock Pro. Start with one capsule, and after one week move to two capsules a day. Use three capsules of Adrenal DMG™ twice today. Take two capsules Stay Young each evening. Now add LivDTox, one capsule a day.

A 2014 study by Danish scientist Dr. Jorn Dyerberg, who first published his work using Eskimo studies, explained that Algae produces a proper ratio of omega fatty acids DHA (70% to EPA (30%) to reduce inflammation and triglycerides. I believe this can help improve the skin. The omega essential fatty acids from Algae are equal to those found in fish oil.

Appendix 7

HORMONAL TESTING AND BALANCE FOR HEALTHY SKIN

Now let's review additional solutions to improve the quality of the skin and one's overall health. *The skin is a reflection of one's overall health because beauty starts from within.* Since many skin issues start with hormonal imbalances, the first step in improving your skin is to go to **GrowYoungand-Slim.com** and take a wellness survey that can help you identify hormonal deficiencies or excesses.

Then request a test kit from our web site www.DelgadoProtocol.com. Click on ALL Products, then click on Hormone Testing Kits. You will be sent the kit with details to measure your hormones by saliva, blood, and/or urine hormones. We can then assist you in determining if you have hormonal imbalances that can cause skin problems like acne. The information below will help you to understand possible solutions to acne.

Saliva

Testosterone, DHT, Androstenedione, Estrone, Estradiol, Estriol, DHEA, Cortisol, (AM) 17-OH, Progesterone, Melatonin

Blood

Female panel: Estradiol, SHBG, E2, DHEA, Progesterone, Cortisol, Free, Total Testosterone with metabolic panel*

Male panel: Free, Total Testosterone, DHT, Estradiol, PSA, SHBG, E2, DHEA, Progesterone, Cortisol, metabolic panel*

Comprehensive Hormone & Metabolic Panel:

- MAJOR HORMONES:
- ANDROGENS: Testosterone & DHT & PSA(male)
- ESTROGENS: Estradiol & Estrone & Estriol (female)
- Progesterone & LH & FSH
- SHBG- Sex Hormone Binding Protein
- Rejuvenation Growth Factors: IGF-1 & IGF-BP3
- ADRENALS: DHEA-S & Cortisol
- INFLAMMATION, DIABETES, IRON
- Hemoglobin A1C, Ferritin (iron) & C-Reactive Protein-CRP,hs
- Vitamin D 25 OH
- Lipid Panel: Cholesterol, HDL, LDL, Ratio HDL/Chol.
- THYROID: TSH &T3, free & T4, free

Metabolic Panel:*

- **Glucose** - Energy source for the body; a steady supply must be available for use, and a relatively constant level of glucose must be maintained in the blood.
- **Calcium** - One of the most important minerals in the body; essential for the proper functioning of muscles,

nerves, and the heart and is required in blood clotting and in the formation of bones

- **Proteins** - Albumin, a small protein produced in the liver; the major protein in serum and total protein, measures albumin as well as all other proteins in serum
- **Electrolytes** - Sodium - Vital to normal body processes, including nerve and muscle function & Potassium - Vital to cell metabolism and muscle function & CO2 (carbon dioxide, bicarbonate) - Helps to maintain the body's acid-base balance (pH) & Chloride - Helps to regulate the amount of fluid in the body and maintain the acid-base balance

Kidney Tests

- BUN (blood urea nitrogen) - Waste product filtered out of the blood by the kidneys; conditions that affect the kidney have the potential to affect the amount of urea in the blood.
- Creatinine - Waste product produced in the muscles; filtered out of the blood by the kidneys so blood levels are a good indication of how well the kidneys are working

Liver Tests

- ALP (alkaline phosphatase) - Enzyme found in the liver and other tissues, bone; elevated levels of ALP in the blood are most commonly caused by liver disease or bone disorders.
- ALT (alanine amino transferase, also called SGPT) - Enzyme found mostly in the cells of the liver and kidney; a useful test for detecting liver damage

- AST (aspartate amino transferase, also called SGOT) - Enzyme found especially in cells in the heart and liver; also a useful test for detecting liver damage
- Bilirubin - Waste product produced by the liver as it breaks down and recycles aged red blood cells

CBC- Complete Blood Count:

- White blood cell count (WBC or Leukocyte count)
- WBC differential count- neutrophils, lymphocytes, basophils, eosinophils, and monocytes.
- Red blood cell count (RBC or erythrocyte count)
- Hematocrit (Hct) & Hemoglobin (Hbg)
- Mean corpuscular volume (MCV)
- Mean corpuscular hemoglobin (MCH)
- Mean corpuscular hemoglobin concentration (MCHC)
- Red cell distribution width (RDW)
- Platelet count
- Mean platelet volume (MPV)

Have hormone testing to improve your skin and the quality of life

We have listed all the most important lab tests for hormones above and the symptom questions at the end of this section to help you and our health coaches or your health care practitioner create a plan to decide which diet, supplements and dosages are best for you.

Complete 24-Hour Urine Steroid Hormone Profile

Includes:

Estrone
 (E1)

2-Hydroxy-estrone
 (2OH-E1)

16a-Hydroxy-estrone
 (16OH-E1)

4-Hydroxy-estrone
 (4OH-E1)

Estradiol
 (E2)

Estriol
 (E3)

Testosterone

Dihydrotestosterone
 (DHT)*

Androstanediol
 (5aAD3a17b)

Androstenedione

Dehydroepiandrosterone
 (DHEA)

Androstenetriol
 (5-AT)

Androsterone
 (AN)

Male Only

11b-hydroxy-Androsterone
 (11bOH-AN)

Etiocholanolone
 (ET)

11b-hydroxy-Etiocholanolone
 (11bOH-ET)

Progesterone

Pregnanediol
 (PD)

5-pregnene-3b,17a,20a-triiol
 (5-PT)

Cortisone (E)

Tetrahydrocortisone
 (THE)

Tetrahydrocorticosterone
 (5a-THB)

Tetrahydro-11-dehydrocorticosterone
 (THA)

Cortisol
 (F)

Tetrahydrocortisol
 (THF)

5a-Tetrahydrocortisol
 (5a-THF)

Lab Tests summary for Acne

It is best to test your hormones by male or female panel, along with a saliva test as your starting point. After you have been put on a plan of personalized supplements, diet and fitness, have your 24 urine test within one month to find out how well your body is absorbing nutrients and what adjustments need to be made to further your progress.

If you budget is limited, then start with the saliva test for hormones. It is the simplest and most affordable way to test 11 important hormones. Saliva is particularly accurate for cortisol and DHEA if you haven't been on hormone therapy, or if you are not currently on birth control pills.

If you are concerned about acne and skin breakouts, we have health educators and doctors who can help you analyze your Androstenedione, testosterone, and DHT levels. This will also tell you if your Estrone levels are higher you're your Estradiol or Estriol levels.

In healthy well-balanced females, Estriol should be higher than Estrone or Estradiol.

If the Estradiol or Estrone levels are high, it is recommended that women start using LivDTox/Cell Stabilizer along with Estro Block® to reduce elevated Estradiol and Estrone levels which contribute to estrogen dominance.

If you have symptoms of estrogen dominance, heavy periods, fibroid growths, endometriosis, belly and excessive hip or breast fat, or breast tumors then look closely for excess levels of estrone and estradiol as compared to estriol and progesterone.

Some women with smaller breasts (a sign of higher androgen and not enough good estrogen (2OHE)), should consider estriol cream if tests indicate there is a need for estrogen. Estriol is a safer estrogen, and some doctors feel it provides more benefit with fewer side effects.

Even gentle estriol cream therapy must still be supported with the use of Estro Block® as well as the addition of Adrenal DMG™ with cortisol support to balance potentially higher DHEA levels. The goal here is to prevent too much Estrone (16aOHE) build up which could be a source indirectly increasing DHT or androstenedione (as explained elsewhere in this book).

The tests to monitor DHT and free testosterone and androstenedione may be the cause of skin breakouts and acne. However, there are more sophisticated tests that can measure enzyme activity directly in the skin, which increases the conversion of hormone metabolites such as DHT, androstenedione, Free Testosterone or Estrone in the skin. These types of tests are only done in research labs.

You may next have the male or female blood panel or for only a few hundred dollars more we do offer a comprehensive metabolic hormone blood panel. With either blood panel we can detect levels of binding proteins includes SHBG. Binding proteins affect the ability of hormones to exert their biological benefit. If the binding proteins are high enough you will have less acne, because the binding proteins tend to reduce acne because fewer androgen hormones are circulating in the general circulation.

If the binding proteins are too high then they attach to the hormones too tightly and create deficiencies. Lower levels of binding proteins are desirable for men and athletes because there are potentially more circulating androgen hormones to improve performance.

We measure insulin because high levels increase risk of acne. We test for lipids which include triglycerides since high levels of fat in the blood cause the insulin to become desensitized which will increase the risk of diabetes, lupus and acne.

Lab tests may be "normal" and your patient may still have acne. The tests in saliva or blood hormones, including high level of androstenedione, high free testosterone, and excess levels of DHEA, excess Estradiol, or excess estrone in saliva or blood all have been found to increase the risk of acne.

Go to DelgadoProtocol.com, click on All Products, then click on Hormone test kits. Get your test kit sent to you. Take the test with the instructions included in the test kit.

Next complete the Hormone Symptom Self-evaluation in the section below, and then note: key guidance you can identify the best supplements and lifestyle steps to improve the quality of your life.

This is a self-scoring test with important questions like "do you have cold hands or feet? Do you have dry skin? Each of the answers to these and other questions can relate to a hormone imbalance or deficiency. We work with or refer to a team of doctors who can help interpret the answers as the compare to the lab test results. The tests for a full thyroid panel can include Free T3, Free T4, Reverse T3, and TSH.

You can also have an iodine test. If low, consider proper natural treatment with iodine as in RAD Iodine™ with an average of 15 mg when taking every other day. Take a compound your doctor suggests or ask about Westhroid that offers a good balance of T3 with T4.

If you doctors has tested you for Thyroid Peroxidase TPO and Thyroglobulin antibodies as positive with Hashimotos or early signs of this more extreme thyroid disorder, you will benefit from closer monitoring by your doctor, and the additions of Vitamin D and T3 – Triiodothyronine, and T4, Thyroxine at optimal dosing

Visit and read the web site **EstroBlock.com** for more detailed solutions. See **AnnihilateAcneNow.com** for additional support and answers to your questions.

Therefore, we like to encourage those with symptoms related to deficiencies or excesses to take a 10 page in depth FREE survey at **www.growyoungandslim.com** under Delgado coaching (see wellness survey the section) or go to DelgadoProtocol.com for the Hormone, Lifestyle assessment.

Hormone Symptom Self Evaluation

Check YES if you have this issue, NO if you do not.

Ask Yourself These Questions: Do you have...	Yes	No
1 Night Sweats, Hot Flashes? Irregular Or Painful Periods?		
2 Forgetful, Poor Memory? Thin Vertical Wrinkles Above Lips?		
3 Acne, Anxiety Attacks? Agitated? Losing Hair Top Head		
4 Frequent Illness, Colds, Flu?		
5 Allergic Reactions, Sneezing, Runny Nose, Sore Throat?		
6 Need 20 Minutes To An Hour Nap To Get Through The Day?		
7 Arthritis Or Inflammatory In Hips, Knees, Hands, Shoulder?		
8 Poor Muscle Tone In Arms And Legs?		
9 Unsatisfactory Outcome Or Body Gains After Long Workouts?		
10 Has Your Sexual Drive Dropped Off Leaving You Frustrated And Hopeless?		
11 Low Libido Or Orgasmic Pleasure?		
12 Do You Have Fat On Your Belly?		
13 Skin Have A Pale Appearance?		
14 Excess Fat In Hips, Thighs, Abdomen? Large Swollen Breast?		
15 Overweight Or Obese Needing To Reduce More Than 50 Lbs.?		
16 Sleep Poorly, Insomnia, Difficult To Return To Sleep, Wake Feeling Tired? Cold hands & feet?		
17 Hypertension, Atherosclerosis, Diabetes, Melanoma, Cancer?		
18 Thinning Hair, Skin, Deep Wrinkled Face?		
19 Sagging Skin Or Under Arm Cellulite?		
20 Difficulty Recovering After Staying Up Late?		

GLOSSARY

A4M-American Academy of Anti-Aging Medicine. See **Worldhealth.net**

Androgens: A group of steroid hormones that stimulate and control anabolic and androgenic characteristics in men and women. The hormones include testosterone, DHT, DHEA, androstenedione, androstenediol, and androsterone.

Beta-sitosterol: A phytochemical, or photosterol found naturally in pecans, avocados, pumpkin seeds, rice bran with a similar structure to cholesterol and known to reduce cholesterol. Cholesterol levels can become elevated in the male prostate, and this ingredient may reduce the size of a swollen prostate. If pregnant, use the ingredient in the lowest dosage to be safe.

Bio-identical hormones are synthesized to be identical to what is found in the human body. These hormones must be taken properly, monitored and used in low dosages in combination with phytochemicals to make their use safer.

The substances in hormone replacement therapy (HRT) are also synthesized. The problem with HRT is that these chemical hormones are altered and slightly different than what is typically in the human body. This can cause dangerous unknown potential side effects.

Cortisol: A natural hormone produced by the adrenal glands to protect the body from stress, inflammation, and disease. This hormone also regulates the release of glucose, free fatty acids, and amino acids. This gives a person a sense of satisfaction upon eating. Low or high levels are of concern. There are tests for saliva, blood, and urine to check on levels and questions to ask regarding fatigue, weight gain or weight loss, flu, cold and arthritis.

DHT: The most dominate androgen and anabolic hormone. This hormone, if elevated in the skin, can increase the likelihood of acne. There are ways to reduce dominate, harmful forms of estrogen which has been recently shown to reduce DHT to safer levels.

DIM-Diindolymethane comes naturally from cruciferous vegetables and in the right concentrations can help reduce body fat, harmful forms of estrogen, and the risk of certain forms of cancer. It has been shown as safe when used with Tamoxifen, a drug used to treat breast cancer. Check with your doctor if you are on drugs that might be affected by DIM. Higher dosages than 600 mg a day (Estro Block Pro® four a day, or Estro Block® six a day) can, in some people, cause temporary side effects like headaches or gastrointestinal distress. Increase your water intake and reduce dosage until symptoms go away.

Estradiol is 10 times more potent than estrone and 80 times more potent than estriol. Estradiol is not as potent as metabolites of estrogen such as 16aOHE or 4Methoxy Estrone. Levels will vary in women depending on the monthly cycle, diet, and supplements. Men exposed to high levels of estradiol develop serious side effects, feminizing, and body fat gain. However, Estradiol in the right balance is essential to good health for men and women.

Free radical damage is oxidative damage to tissues from single unpaired electrons. In high levels, aging and disease proceeds faster. Anti-oxidants such as transdermal melatonin, nitric oxide from nitrate plants such as kale, beets, Swiss chard, and a diet low in animal based products, more of a plant-based diet, reduces free radical damage. Exercise initially increases free radical damage. As your body adjusts, the free radicals clear faster.

Indole 3-Cabinol (I3C) comes from natural cruciferous vegetables, improves estrogen metabolism, and may reduce certain forms of cancer and acne. Works well at lower dosages with DIM.

IGF-1, an insulin-like growth factor, is a protein produced by the liver to stimulate body tissue growth, muscle, liver, skin, lungs.

Methyl-donors such as DMG or TMG and 5MTHF help the body to improve biochemical processes. This improves liver function and the body's ability to produce energy.

Progesterone is a hormone critical to the female cycle. Progesterone levels are relatively low during the preovulatory phase of the menstrual cycle, rise after ovulation, and are elevated during the luteal phase. Women with chronic low levels may resort to nicotine, alcohol, and marijuana to enhance serotonin levels. Progesterone may reduce cravings.

SHBG is produced in the liver and transports most of the major sex hormones in the blood. It binds tightly to testosterone, DHT, androstenediol, estradiol and estrone. It is weakly bound to DHEA and androstenedione. SHBG levels are *decreased* by androgens, administration of anabolic steroids, polycystic ovary syndrome POCS, hypothyroidism, diabetes, obesity, Cushing's Syndrome, and acromegaly. SHBG levels *increase* with estrogenic states (oral contraceptives), pregnancy, hyperthyroidism, cirrhosis, anorexia nervosa, and certain drugs. Long-term calorie restriction of more than 50 percent increases SHBG, while lowering free and total testosterone and estradiol.

Spirolactone-aldactone is typically used for high blood pressure or heart failure and sometimes used to treat acne, with side effects of cramps, chest pain, coma, confusion, constipation, cough, diarrhea, dizziness, hives, itching, loss of appetite, skin rash, bleeding, vomiting of blood, yellow eyes, or skin.

Xenoestrogens are a type of xenohormone (BPA, Dioxin, Phthalates in perfumes, cosmetics, methylparaben) that imitates estrogen. They can be either synthetic or natural chemical compounds. Synthetic xenoestrogens are widely used in industrial compounds, such as PCBs, BPA and phthalates (feminizing chemicals on male development) precocious puberty in eight or nine year olds has been linked to exposure to exogenous estrogenic compounds.

BEST BOOKS & WEBSITES

Supplements:
DelgadoProtocol.com

Whole super foods diet:
Simply Healthy by Nick Delgado, PhD
Going Raw, Judita Wignail
The China Study by T. Colin Campbell, PhD
The Starch Solution by John McDougall, MD

Fitness:
Stay Young by Nick Delgado, PhD
Eat & Run by Scott Jurek

Hormone Balance:
Grow Young and Slim by Nick Delgado, PhD
Hormone Solution by Thierry Hertoghe, MD
Stay Young & Sexy by Jonathan Wright, MD
I'm Too Young for This! Suzanne Somers
Growyoungandslim.com, *Anti-Aging Make Over*
Estroblock.com
NickDelgado.com
AnnihilateAcneNow.com membership site for support

Power of mind:

Growyoungandslim.com motivation

LFC glasses (Laser Focus Concentration)

NickDelgadoevents.com

Supreme Influence by Niurka

REFERENCES

Books/eBooks

Grow Young and Slim by Nick Delgado

http://www.antiagingage.com/pdf/ebook_Grow-Young-and-Slim.pdf

The Hormone Handbook. Thierry Hertoghe / Bombshell by Suzanne Somers Acne for Dummies**

http://books.google.com/books?id=s44M16iKQXMC&pg=PT86&lpg=PT86&dq=androstenedione+acne&source=bl&ots=1sK6ySVBat&sig=VyWDnk5BkdjcUo2FLABzZBXqqb8&hl=en&sa=X&ei=LWgUU9yRDNHtoAT7-oCAAg&ved=0CEgQ6AEwAw#v=onepage&q=androstenedione%20acne&f=false

Youtube.com

Birth control pills and acne

https://www.youtube.com/watch?v=IzkNpJLHoE8

Web sites

http://www.ncbi.nlm.nih.gov/pmc/articles/PMC2923944/

http://www.anapsid.org/cnd/hormones/estrogen.html

http://www.drmcdougall.com/health/education/health-science/common-health-problems/acne/

Acne Has Nothing to Do with Diet – Wrong!
http://www.nealhendrickson.com/mcdougall/031100puacne.htm

The Fat Vegan
http://www.drmcdougall.com/misc/2008nl/dec/fat.htm

Vitamin B5, DHEA for Lupus

http://jeffreydachmd.com/

http://www.healthywomen.org/glossary/term/5543

http://www.drnorthrup.com/womenshealth/healthcenter/topic_det
ails.php?topic_id=55

http://www.yourhormones.info/hormones/androstenedione.aspx

http://www.wholehealthchicago.com/3376/diindolylmethance-
dim/

Androstenedione - Why the oral supplement is bad for the skin
http://www.gettingfit.com/andro.html

What patients are saying about Androstenedione and Acne
http://treato.com/Androstenedione,Acne/?a=s&p=6

Androgen Excess

Author: Mohamed Yahya Abdel-Rahman, MD, MSc; Chief Editor:
Richard Scott Lucidi, MD Updated: Aug 7, 2012

Louann Brizendine, M.D. - 2007 - *Science*. In a study at the University of Utah, the most in-your-face aggressive teenage girls were found to have high levels of the androgen *androstenedione*. High level of androstenedione was found to cause acne. With high inhibitor concentrations >10 M, metabolite formation was consistently re-

duced to undetectable levels.
http://dmd.aspetjournals.org/content/25/7/853.full

How DIM works explained biochemically,
http://examine.com/supplements/Diindolylmethane/

Journals:

Abraham GE: "Ovarian and adrenal contribution to peripheral androgens during the menstrual cycle." *J Clin Endocrinol Metab* 1974; 39: 340-346.

Arukwe A, Celius T, Walther BT, Goksøyr A (June 2000). "Effects of xenoestrogen treatment on zona radiata protein and vitellogenin expression in Atlantic salmon (Salmo salar)." *Aquat. Toxicol.* **49** (3): 159–170. doi:10.1016/S0166-445X(99)00083-1. PMID 10856602.

Bagga D, Ashley JM, Geffrey SP, Wang HJ, Barnard RJ, Korenman S, Heber D. *Cancer.* 1995 Dec 15;76(12):2491-6.

Bagga D, Ashley JM, Geffrey SP, Wang HJ, Barnard RJ, Korenman S, Heber D. *Cancer.* 1995 Dec 15;76(12):2491-6.

Betti R, Bencini PL, Lodi A, Urbani CE "Incidence of Polycystic Ovaries in Patients with Late-Onset or Persistent Acne: Hormonal Reports" *Dermatology* Vol. 181, No. 2, 1990
http://www.karger.com/Article/Abstract/247896
Summary: Among the acne patients, the women with ovarian abnormalities had higher values of androstenedione, dehydroepiandrosterone, dehydroepiandrosterone sulfate and luteinizing hormone (LH) and a higher LHT/follicle-stimulating hormone ratio than those with acne and without ovarian abnormalities.
http://www.sciencedirect.com/science/article/pii/S001078249900093
1
Contraception Volume 60, Issue 5, November 1999, Pages 255–262

Buterin T, Koch C, Naegeli H (August 2006). "Convergent transcriptional profiles induced by endogenous estrogen and distinct xenoestrogens in breast cancer cells." *Carcinogenesis* **27** (8): 1567–78. doi:10.1093/carcin/bgi339. PMID 16474171.

Cela E, Robertson C, Rush K, Kousta E, White DM, Wilson H, Lyons G, Kingsley P, McCarthy MI and Franks S "Prevalence of polycystic ovaries in women with androgenic alopecia." *Department of Obstetrics and Gynaecology,* St Mary's Hospital, London W2 1PG, Hammersmith Hospital, London W12 0NN, UK.

Cordain L. "Acne vulgaris: a disease of Western civilization." *Arch Dermatol.* 2002 Dec; 138(12):1584-90.

D'Amato et al (1994) "2-Methoxyestradiol, an endogenous mammalian metabolite, inhibits tubulin polymerization by interacting at the colchicine site." *Proc.Natl.Acad.Sci.U.S.A.* 91 3964. PMID: 8171020.

Dallinga JW, Moonen EJ, Dumoulin JC, Evers JL, Geraedts JP, Kleinjans JC (August 2002). "Decreased human semen quality and organochlorine compounds in blood." *Hum. Reprod.* **17** (8): 1973–9. doi:10.1093/humrep/17.8.1973. PMID 12151423.

Darbre PD (March 2006). "Environmental oestrogens, cosmetics and breast cancer." *Best Pract. Res. Clin. Endocrinol. Metab.* **20** (1): 121–43. doi:10.1016/j.beem.2005.09.007. PMID 16522524.

Darbre PD, Aljarrah A, Miller WR, Coldham NG, Sauer MJ, Pope GS (2004). "Concentrations of parabens in human breast tumours." *J Appl Toxicol* **24** (1): 5–13. doi:10.1002/jat.958. PMID 14745841.

Falsetti L, Ramazzotto Francesca, Rosina Barbara, "Efficacy of combined ethinyloestradiol (0.035 mg) and cyproterone acetate (2 mg) in acne and hirsutism in women with polycystic ovary syndrome of Obstetrics & 1997" - informahealthcare.com 1997, Vol. 17, No. 6 , Pages 565-568

Forstrom L, Mustakallio KK, Dessypris A, Uggeldahl PE, Adlecrutz H: "Plasma testosterone levels and acne." *Acta Derm Venereol* (Stockh) 1974; 54: 369371.

Frommer D, "Changing Age of the Menopause," *Br Med J 2* (1964):349

Fulton JE Jr. "Effect of chocolate on acne vulgaris" *JAMA.* 1969 Dec 15; 210(11):2071-4.

Gilliland JM, Kirk J, Smeaton TC: "Normalized androgen ratio: Its application to clinical dermatology." *Clin Exp Dermatol* 1981; 6: 349-353.

Golden RJ, Noller KL, Titus-Ernstoff L, Kaufman RH, Mittendorf R, Stillman R, Reese EA (March 1998). "Environmental endocrine modulators and human health: an assessment of the biological evidence." *Crit. Rev. Toxicol.* **28** (2): 109–227.doi:10.1080/10408449891344191. PMID 9557209.

Greenwalt, David, androstenedione specialist, in an interview in *Muscle and Fitness,* July, 1998.

Hatwal A, Bhatt RP, Agrawal JK, Singh G, Bajpai HS: "Spironolactone and cimetidine in treatment of acne." *Acta Derm Venereol* (Stockh) 1988; 68:84-87.

Hatwal A, Singh SK, Agarwal JK, Singh G, Bajpai HS, Gupta SS *Serum testosterone, DHEA-S and androstenedione levels in acne* 1990 Volume 56 Issue 6 Page 427-429

Hay JB, Hodgins MB: "Metabolism of androgens in human skin in acne." *Brit J Dermatol* 1974; 91: 123133.

Hazeldinea Jon, Wiebke Arltb, Lord Janet M. "Dehydroepiandrosterone as a regulator of immune cell function," *The Journal of*

Steroid Biochemistry and Molecular Biology Volume 120, Issues 2–3, 31 May 2010, Pages 127–136

Hoehn GH. "Acne and diet." *Cutis.* 1966; 2:389-94.

Inclendon Thomas RD, Director of Sports Nutrition, Human Performance Specialists, Inc. via e-mail, 2000. *J Amer Med Assoc,* "Oral Androstenedione Administration and Serum Testosterone Concentrations in Young Men" 2000; 283:779-782.

Kagawa Y, "Impact of Westernization on the Nutrition of Japanese: Changes in Physique, Cancer, Longevity, and Centenarians," *Prev Med 7* (1978):205

Karrer-Voegeli S1, Rey F, Reymond MJ, Meuwly JY, Gaillard RC, Gomez F. "Androgen dependence of hirsutism, acne, and alopecia in women: retrospective analysis of 228 patients investigated for hyperandrogenism." *Medicine* (Baltimore). 2009 Jan; 88(1):32-45.doi: 10.1097/md.0b013e3181946a2c.
http://www.ncbi.nlm.nih.gov/pubmed/19352298
"Anabolic Steroids in Sport and Exercise, Human Kinetics," 1993. *J Amer Med Assoc,* 1999; 281:2020-2028.

King, et al. "Effect of oral androstenedione on serum testosterone and adaptations to resistance training in young men." *J Amer Med Assoc,* 1999; 281:2020-2028.

Kligman AM: "An overview of acne." *J Invest Dermatol* 1974; 62: 268-287.

Kuo P. "The effect of lipemia upon coronary and peripheral arterial circulation in patients with essential hyperlipemia." *Am J Med.* 1959 Jan; 26(1):68-75

Kuttenn Frédérique, Mowszowicz Iréne, Schaison Gilbert and Pierre Mauvais-Jarvis "Androgen Production and Skin Metabolism

In Hirsutism"
http://joe.endocrinology-journals.org/content/75/1/83.short
Summary: These results indicate that androstenedione is the principal androgen secreted in hirsutism. The high rate of excretion of androstanediol in the urine of patients with idiopathic hirsutism may be explained by the fact that this steroid is an end-product of testosterone metabolism.

LaVallee et al (2002) "2-Methoxyestradiol inhibits proliferation and induces apoptosis independently of estrogen receptors α and β." *Cancer Res.* 62 3691. PMID: 12097276.

LaVallee et al (2003) "2-Methoxyestradiol up-regulates death receptor 5 and induces apoptosis through activation of the extrinsic pathway." *Cancer Res.* 63 468. PMID: 12543804.

Levell[1] MJ[*], Cawood[1] ML, Burke[2] B, Cunliffe[2] WJ "Acne is not associatedwith abnormal plasma androgens" *British Journal of Dermatology* Volume 120, Issue 5, pages 649–654, May 1989

Li DK, Zhou Z, Miao M, He Y, Wang J, Ferber J, Herrinton LJ, Gao E, Yuan W (February 2011). "Urine bisphenol-A (BPA) level in relation to semen quality." *Fertil. Steril.* **95** (2): 625–30.e1–4. doi:10.1016/j.fertnstert.2010.09.026. PMID 21035116.

Lim JS, James VHT: "Plasma androgens in acne vulgaris." *Brit J Dermatol* 1974; 91: 135-143.

Logan AC. "Omega-3 fatty acids and acne." *Arch Dermatol.* 2003 Jul; 139(7):941-2;

Lucky AW, McGuire J, Rosenfeld RL, Lucky PA, Rich BH: "Plasma androgens in women with acne vulgaris." *J Invest Dermatol* 1983; 81: 70-74.

Marynick SP, Chakmajian ZH, McCaffree DL, C Herndon JH: "Androgen excess in cystic acne." *N Engl J Med* 1983; 308: 981-986.

Mendoza SG, Zerpa A, Carrasco H, et al. "Estradiol, testosterone, apolipoproteins, lipoprotein cholesterol, and lipolytic enzymes in men with premature myocardial infarction and angiographically assessed coronary occlusion." *Artery.*1983; 12:1-23.

Michaelsson G. "Diet and acne" *Nutr Rev.* 1981 Feb; 39(2):104-6.

Morishima A, Grumbach M M, Simpson E R, Fisher C, and Qin K. *Aromatase deficiency in male and female siblings caused by a novel mutation and the physiological role of estrogens.* DOI: **http://dx.doi.org/10.1210/jcem.80.12.8530621** Published Online: July 01, 2013

Murray DW, Lichter SR (April 1998). "Organochlorine residues and breast cancer." *N. Engl. J. Med.* **338** (14): 990–1.PMID 9527611.

Olea N, Olea-Serrano F, Lardelli-Claret P, Rivas A, Barba-Navarro A (1999). "Inadvertent exposure to xenoestrogens in children." *Toxicol Ind Health* **15** (1–2): 151–8. doi:10.1177/074823379901500112. PMID 10188197.

Palmlund I (June 1996). "Exposure to a xenoestrogen before birth: the diethylstilbestrol experience." *J Psychosom Obstet Gynaecol* **17** (2): 71–84. doi:10.3109/01674829609025667. PMID 8819018.

Price Vera H, MD, FRCP(C) "Testosterone Metabolism in the Skin: A Review of Its Function in Androgenetic Alopecia, Acne Vulgaris, and Idiopathic Hirsutism Including Recent Studies With Anti-androgens" *Arch Dermatol.* 1975; 111(11):1496-1502. doi:10.1001/archderm.1975
Summary: a temporary, increased dihydrotestosterone formation at specific skin target sites at different ages causes the normal devel-

opment of certain sexual characteristics, as well as the androgen dependent skin disorders.

Pugazhendhi D, Sadler AJ, Darbre PD (2007). "Comparison of the
global gene expression profiles produced by methylparaben, n-
butylparaben and 17beta-oestradiol in MCF7 human breast cancer
cells." *J Appl Toxicol* **27** (1): 67–77. doi:10.1002/jat.1200.PMID
17121429.

Rasmussen JE. "Diet and acne" *Int J Dermatol.* 1977 Jul-Aug;
16(6):488-92.

Rim SJ. "Decrease in coronary blood flow reserve during hyper-
lipidemia is secondary to an increase in blood viscosity." *Circulation.*
2001 Nov 27, 04(22):2704-9.

**Roberts CK, Barnard RJ, Sindhu RK, Jurczak M, Ehdaie A, Vaziri
ND.** *J Appl Physiol* (1985). 2005 Jan; 98(1):203-10. Epub 2004 Aug
27.PMID: 15333612 [PubMed – indexed for MEDLINE] Free Article.
Select item 6827033

Roberts CK, Vaziri ND, Sindhu RK, Barnard RJ. *J Appl Physiol*
(1985). 2003 Mar;94(3):941-6. Epub 2002 Oct 25.

Rogan WJ, Ragan NB (July 2003). "Evidence of effects of environmental chemicals on the endocrine system in children."*Pediatrics* **112**
(1 Pt 2): 247–52. doi:10.1542/peds.112.1.S1.247. PMID 12837917.

Rosenberg EW. "Acne diet reconsidered." *Arch Dermatol.* 1981 Apr;
117(4):193-5.

Safe S (December 2004). "Endocrine disruptors and human health:
is there a problem." *Toxicology* **205** (1–2): 3–10.
doi:10.1016/j.tox.2004.06.032. PMID 15458784.

Sansone, Gail; Reisner, Ronald M "Differential rates of conversion of testerone to dihydrotestosterone in acne and in normal human skin- a possible pathogenic factor in acne." *Journal of Investigative Dermatology.* May71, 1971 Vol. 56 Issue 5, p366-372. 7p
Summary: Acne bearing skin produced from 2 to 20 times more dihydrotestosterone than normal back skin.
http://www.eje-online.org/content/149/5/439.short

Sansone G, Reisner RM: "Differential rates of conversion of testosterone and dihydrotestosterone in acne and in normal skin: A possible pathogenic factor in acne." *J Invest Dermatol* 1972; 56: 366372.

Schiavone FE, Reitschel RL, Sgontas D, Harris R: "Elevated free testosterone levels in women with acne." *Arch Dermatol* 1983; 119: 799-802.

Sharpe RM, Skakkebaek NE (May 1993). "Are oestrogens involved in falling sperm counts and disorders of the male reproductive tract?" *Lancet* **341** (8857): 1392–5. doi:10.1016/0140-6736(93)90953-E. PMID 8098802.

Sharpe RM (February 2003). "The 'oestrogen hypothesis'- where do we stand now?" *Int. J. Androl.* **26** (1): 2–15. doi:10.1046/j.1365-2605.2003.00367.x. PMID 12534932.

Shaw JC, Expert opinion on pharmacotherapy, 2002 - informahealthcare.com
Summary: Prednisone five – 10 mg nightly or dexamethasone 0.25 – 0.5 mg nightly causes a suppression of ... ACTH release and has been shown to reduce circulating androgens and improve acne [49].The low dose may not cause complete adrenal axis suppression but patients should be.
http://link.springer.com/chapter/10.1007/978-1-4612-2332-0_54
Hormonal therapies in acne July 2002, Vol. 3, No. 7, Pages 865-874

Shimada et al (2003) "Roles of p38 and c-jun NH2-terminal kinase-mediated pathways in 2-methoxyestradiol-induced p53 induction and apoptosis." *Carcinogenesis* 24 1067. PMID: 12807754.

Stanczyk Frank Z, ET. "Androgens, PSA, Finasteride, in men Prostate Cancer risk." Men put on Finasteride, After three to six months, PSA dropped 40%, DHT, and 3 adiol fell 80%, Testosterone levels increased 22 to 28% Hormonal therapies in acne

Strauss JS: "Sebaceous glands: in Dermatology in General Medicine." **Ed Fitzpatrick TB, Eisen AZ, Wolff K, Freedberg IM and Austen KF** *McGrawHill*, USA, 1979.

The Coronary Drug Project Research Group. "The Coronary Drug Project: findings leading to discontinuation of the 2.5-mg/day estrogen group." *J Amer Med Assoc.*1973; 226:652-657.

Thiboutot DM. "Diet and acne revisited." *Arch Dermatol.* 2002 Dec; 138(12):1591-2.

Thiboutot Diane, MD, Gollnick Harald, MD, Bettoli Vincenzo, MD "New insights into the management of acne: An update from the Global Alliance to Improve Outcomes in Acne Group" Journal of the American Academy of Dermatology Volume 60, Issue 5, Supplement 1, Pages S1–S50, May 2009

Tymchuk CN, Tessler SB, Aronson WJ, Barnard RJ. *Nutr Cancer.* 1998;31(2):127-31.

Tymchuk CN, Tessler SB, Barnard RJ. *Nutr Cancer.* 2000;38(2):158-62.

Tymchuk CN, Tessler SB, Aronson WJ, Barnard RJ. *Nutr Cancer.* 1998;31(2):127-31.

Vajda AM, Barber LB, Gray JL, Lopez EM, Woodling JD, Norris DO (May 2008). "Reproductive disruption in fish downstream from an estrogenic wastewater effluent." *Environ. Sci. Technol.* **42** (9): 3407–14. doi:10.1021/es0720661.PMID 18522126.

Walton S, Cunliffe WJ, "Clinical, ultrasound and hormonal markers of androgenicity in acne vulgaris" *British Journal of Dermatology* Volume 133, Issue 2, pages 249–253, August 1995-
Summary: best model for predicting ACNE score as involving Androstendione- DELTA 4 and DHEAS (positive effects), and SHBG (negative effect), $P < 0.005$, $R^2 = 0.36$). In none of the patients were the levels of DHEAS or SHBG outside the normal range

William F, Danby, M "Nutrition and acne Clinics" *Dermatology* Volume 28, Issue 6, November–December 2010, Pages 598–604 Volume 28, Issue 6, November–December 2010, Pages 598–604
http://www.sciencedirect.com/science/article/pii/S0738081X10000416?np=y
Abstract: There are significant data supporting the role of diet in acne. Our Western diet includes many dairy sources containing hormones...both of which promote increased production of available androgens and the subsequent development of acne.

Williams DE, Lech JJ, Buhler DR (March 1998). "Xenobiotics and xenoestrogens in fish: modulation of cytochrome P450 and carcinogenesis." *Mutat. Res.* **399** (2): 179–92. doi:10.1016/S0027-5107(97)00255-8. PMID 9672659.

Zsarnovszky A, Le HH, Wang HS, Belcher SM (December 2005). "Ontogeny of rapid estrogen-mediated extracellular signal-regulated kinase signaling in the rat cerebellar cortex: potent nongenomic agonist and endocrine disrupting activity of the xenoestrogen bisphenol A." *Endocrinology* **146** (12): 5388–96. doi:10.1210/en.2005-0565. PMID 16123166.